Essent

RESEARCH METHODOLOGY

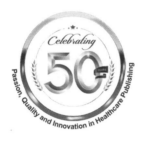

Essentials of
RESEARCH METHODOLOGY
(for all Physiotherapy and Allied Health Sciences Students)

A Thangamani Ramalingam PT MSc (Psy) PGDRM ACS

Edited by
SN Senthil Kumar MSc PT (UK)

JAYPEE BROTHERS MEDICAL PUBLISHERS
The Health Sciences Publisher
New Delhi | London | Panama

Jaypee Brothers Medical Publishers (P) Ltd

Headquarters

Jaypee Brothers Medical Publishers (P) Ltd
4838/24, Ansari Road, Daryaganj
New Delhi 110 002, India
Phone: +91-11-43574357
Fax: +91-11-43574314
Email: jaypee@jaypeebrothers.com

Overseas Offices

J.P. Medical Ltd
83 Victoria Street, London
SW1H 0HW (UK)
Phone: +44 20 3170 8910
Fax: +44 (0)20 3008 6180
Email: info@jpmedpub.com

Jaypee-Highlights Medical Publishers Inc
City of Knowledge, Bld. 235, 2nd Floor
Clayton, Panama City, Panama
Phone: +1 507-301-0496
Fax: +1 507-301-0499
Email: cservice@jphmedical.com

Jaypee Brothers Medical Publishers (P) Ltd
Bhotahity, Kathmandu, Nepal
Phone: +977-9741283608
Email: kathmandu@jaypeebrothers.com

Website: www.jaypeebrothers.com
Website: www.jaypeedigital.com

Essentials of Research Methodology
(for all Physiotherapy and Allied Health Sciences Students)

First Edition: **2019**

ISBN 978-93-5270-609-9

Printed at Rajkamal Electric Press, Kundli, Haryana.

Dedicated to

Late Secretary

MM Amla Sir

Preface

The aim of this book is to help the physiotherapy and allied health sciences students to have an insight regarding the subject matter of research which is commonly felt as a difficult concept as it involves mathematics for academic students and practitioners. It is the responsibility of everyone in the allied health field to update the knowledge of understanding research to contribute to the care of patients as professionals take greater professional responsibility and accountability in the changing scenario of health care.

With two decades of teaching and clinical experience, we have written this book to relieve the allied health sciences students from the anxiety to write down notes. This book is an attempt to make the subject easy and comprehensible to the students also keeping in mind the exam-related need of students. Moreover, as this subject has got many branches and equally good number of books, collecting the information and material needed for the students are very difficult, according to their syllabus. Because of this problem, we have humbly tried to favor students in this regard by writing this book.

The book consists of three parts: Part 1—Introduction to Research; Part 2—Basic Statistics in Research; Part 3—Understanding and Publishing Research; Appendix with Question Bank and Glossary. It has 28 chapters which almost covers the syllabus in any Indian university for "Research" subject in physiotherapy and allied health sciences. It includes special and exclusive topics like psychometric properties of tools, evidence-based physiotherapy, interpretation of statistics, understanding a research article, and critical appraisal of clinical trials.

After listening to voices of students and teachers during our meet with them in different forums and platforms, we understood that there is a need for a book of this type which would highly benefit students of various healthcare disciplines, both undergraduates and postgraduates. Our strong contention is that there is a need for simple, easily understandable textbook on this very hard subject for the above-mentioned student groups. In addition, since high quality clinical research in the above-mentioned disciplines is still far from reality, this book will also cater to the needs of the clinical professionals alike and is expected to serve as a good reference book for them.

After our review on the existing textbooks on the subject, from our understanding, though there are many books available in the academic collections on Research Methodology, on various counts, there is a need for this type of book and we expect that this book would surpass the expectations of the target populations for the following reasons.

Firstly, the simplicity of the language that we have used in the book, examples used and related contents is one main reason why this book would be a favored textbook among student population. We have wide experience in teaching physiotherapy students understand the clear learning need of the students especially the language that should be used for students. Every care has been taken keeping this thought in mind during the preparation of this book. We are confident that this would definitely be an advantage for this book compared to other books available in related titles.

Secondly, we have covered almost most of the topics included in any book on research and biostatistics. Our review of the available books in the market shows that there is a lacuna in every book in terms of the topics covered. No other book has covered all the topics in research methodology and biostatistics like this book has done, especially for the target population of professionals in allied health sciences. We expect that this book is prepared in a simple language on this hard subject. The contents are highlighted; important formulas are boxed making reading and connecting points easy. We expect that this book would benefit other related disciplines in therapeutics and allied health like pharmacy, occupational therapy, speech and language therapy, and nursing.

We have a separately devoted topic on appraisal of research articles, wherein, apart from conducting research process, this book has gone to the next stage of analyzing the research article.

In addition, we have prepared an algorithm on the research process commonly followed in various therapeutic research designs. For a novice researcher, this would be an effective self-guiding and learning tool. When a student or any other clinical person involved in research is dumb stuck in his/her pathway through research process, this algorithm will act as a signpost for making his/her work in an effective manner. Thoughts have gone while writing this book into the scenarios that healthcare professionals encounter into discussion in research topics both at classroom as student and as clinician.

Although we have taken great care in writing this book, but it is possible that we might have committed some errors. Hence, comments and criticism from teachers and students will therefore be highly appreciated and will be rectified in subsequent editions.

Wish you a happy reading.

A Thangamani Ramalingam
SN Senthil Kumar

Acknowledgments

It would be humanly impossible to me to acknowledge all of many people who have given me inspiration and contribution in the writing of this book *Essentials of Research Methodology* in the field of physiotherapy and allied health sciences. It is my pleasure and privilege to engrave the deep sense of gratitude to my teachers who induced a great desire for teaching in me. Words are not enough to express my gratitude to my friend (Mr SN Senthil Kumar), who provided an excellent editorial service.

My thanks also go to the management of Sarvajanik Medical Trust, who accommodated me as teacher and given me all the freedom to accomplish my goal constructively and effectively. I am also extremely grateful to my parents, wife, and my children for their patience and support in writing this book. Moreover, I am equally thankful to my colleagues and friends, for their clean criticism and contributions.

I am thankful to Shri Jitendar P Vij (Group Chairman), Mr Ankit Vij (Managing Director), Mr MS Mani (Group President), Ms Pooja Bhandari (Production Head), Ms Sunita Katla (Executive Assistant to Group Chairman and Publishing Manager), Mr Rajesh Sharma (Production Coordinator), Mr Sharad Patel (Ahmedabad Branch), and team members of M/s Jaypee Brothers Medical Publishers (P) Ltd, New Delhi, India, for all their support to work in this project.

At last my sincere thanks to all the authors who have already worked in this area and helped me in many, many subtle ways.

Syllabus

Introduction to Research Methodology
Meaning of research, objectives of research, motivation in research, types of research and research approaches, research methods vs. methodology, criteria for good research.

Research in Physiotherapy
Introduction, research for physiotherapist: Why? How? and When? Research—definition, concept, purpose, approaches, Internet sites for physiotherapist.

Research Problem
What is a research problem? Statement of research problem, statement of purpose and objectives of research problem, necessity of defining the problem.

Review of Literature
Purpose of review of literature, the process of review of literature, sources of review of literature, strategies for review of literature and principles of writing literature review.

Research Proposal
Research proposal steps and format.

Ethics in Research
Importance of ethics in research, ethical issues in human subjects' research, ethical principles that govern research with human subjects, components of an ethically valid informed consent for research.

Research Design
Meaning of research design, need for research design, features for good design, different research designs, basic principles of research design. Qualitative and quantitative research designs—difference between qualitative and quantitative designs.

Sampling Design
The criteria for selecting sampling procedure, implications for sample design, steps in sampling design, characteristics of good sample

design, different types of sample design, need for sampling and some fundamental definitions, important sampling distributions, standard error and Type I and II error. Population and sample, definition of population and sample, types of sampling, sample size determination and rationale.

Non-probability sampling: Convenience sampling, quota sampling, purposive sampling, advantages and disadvantages of non-probability sampling.

Probability sampling: Simple random sampling, stratified random sampling. Cluster sampling, systematic sampling, advantages and disadvantages of probability sampling.

Measurement and Scaling Techniques and Methods of Data Collection

Measurement in research, measurement scales, sources of error in measurement, technique of developing measurement tools, meaning of scaling, its classification and important scaling techniques. Research reliability, validity and criteria for assessing the measuring the tools. The collection of primary data, collection data through questionnaires and schedules, difference between questionnaires and schedules.

Non-experimental and Experimental Research

Experimental design: Controlled trials, Parallel or concurrent controls, Randomized, Non-randomized, Sequential controls- Self- controlled, Cross over and External controls. Quasi experimental research-advantages and disadvantages of quasi experiments.

Non-experimental design: Observational study design, descriptive or case series, case control studies (retrospective), cross-sectional studies, surveys, cohort studies (prospective) and historical cohort studies.

Processing and Analysis of Data

Processing operations, problems in processing, types of analysis, statistics in research, measures of central tendency, dispersion, asymmetry, relationship. Basic principles of graphical representation, types of diagrams—histograms, frequency polygons, smooth frequency polygon, cumulative frequency curve, normal probability curve.

Measures of Central Tendency—Mean, Median and Mode

Measures of dispersion—range, interquartile range, quartile deviation, mean deviation, standard deviation, coefficient deviation.

Testing of Hypothesis

What is hypothesis? Basic concepts concerning testing of hypothesis, procedure of hypothesis testing, measuring the power of hypothesis test, tests of hypothesis, limitations of the tests of hypothesis: (a) Null hypothesis; (b) Alternative hypothesis; (c) Acceptance and rejection of null hypothesis; (d) Level of significance.

Parametric and Nonparametric Tests

(a) Chi square test; (b) Mann-Whitney U test; (c) Wilcoxon Signed test; (d) Kruskal-Wallis test; (e) Friedman test; (f) t-test/student t test; (g) Analysis of variance; (h) Standard errors of differences.

Reporting Research

(a) Writing the report; (b) Documentation; (c) Details of the study; (d) Arrangement of report; (e) Practice—presentation of study for discussion; (f) Method of teaching—lecture and discussion—seminars and practices; how and what to read from journals?

Writing Research for Publication

Guidelines to publish a research paper and its contents.

Introduction to Statistics

Meaning, definition, characteristics of statistics. Importance of the study of statistics, branches of statistics, statistics and health science including physiotherapy, parameters and estimates, descriptive and inferential statistics, variables and their types, measurement scales.

Correlation and Regression

Correlation—meaning, types of correlation, scatter diagram, Karl Pearson's coefficient of correlation, Spearman's rank correlation, coefficient. Logistic regression and multiple linear regression, regression coefficient.

Analysis of Variance and Covariance

Analysis of variance (ANOVA), basic principles of ANOVA, ANOVA technique; analysis of covariance (ANCOVA).

Interpretation of Statistical Results

Interpreting significant and non-significant results, discussion and conclusion of obtained results, guidelines to interpret and critique research results.

Contents

Fundamentals of Research

+ Introduction to Research
+ Research in Physiotherapy
+ Research Process
+ Research Problem and Literature Review
+ Research Design
+ Sampling Design and Sampling Distributions
+ Measurement, Scaling, Data Collection and Processing
+ Ethics in Research
+ Research Reporting
+ Experimental and Non-Experimental Research Designs
+ Analysis of Variance Study (ANOVA) Designs
+ Pilot Study in Research
+ Psychometric Properties of Tools
+ Qualitative Research
+ Survey Research

Fundamentals of Research

Introduction to Research

INTRODUCTION

Evolving nature of science aims towards reliable information about human health for understanding the disease process and its development to prevent and treat the sufferers. The only way to gather the essential information is research which uses scientific methods for obtaining that information. Though various types of research methods are being followed, the aim of this text is to introduce the readers various types of scientific research and scientific methods.

Science and Scientific Method

Science refers to a system of acquiring knowledge. This is a rigorous system which uses observation and experimentation to describe and explain natural phenomena. It can be said that it is a search towards the explanation of truth behind a subject or phenomenon. Hence, the term science refers to the organized body of knowledge people have gained using that system. Though there are benefits with scientific system of gaining knowledge it is equally meted with difficulties which can be termed as limitations of this method.

Limitations of Scientific Method

1. Problems of collection of data and conceptualization may occur.
2. Repetition problems.
3. Outdated and insufficient information system may cause problems.
4. Sometimes lack of resources becomes an obstacle.

5. Non-availability of trained researchers.
6. Absence of code of conduct.

Every aspect of human learning and evolution has been through search for truth behind our existence otherwise termed as "Research". The word research is derived from the Middle French "*recherche*", which means "to go about seeking". The earliest recorded use of the term was in 1577. Though it covers every aspect of human learning, Research in general is the process of finding the solution for the raised question in each defined area. Thus this piling up new information to understand the true nature of a being has been defined in many ways.

DEFINITIONS

Research has been defined in a number of different ways. The following are the few definitions:

"In the broadest sense of the word, the definition of research includes any gathering of data, information and facts for the advancement of knowledge". — *Martyn Shuttleworth*

"Research is a process of steps used to collect and analyze information to increase our understanding of a topic or issue".
— *Creswell*

"A systematic investigation, including research development, testing and evaluation, designed to develop or contribute to generalizable knowledge".

Webster Dictionary defines research in more detail as *"a studious inquiry or examination".*

CHARACTERISTICS OF RESEARCH

Scientific research exhibits some characteristics
- Research is logical and objective.
- It is a search for knowledge.
- Research is Empirical and Systematic and is based on the scientific method.
- It finds out relationship between two or more variables.
- All variables are controlled except those that are experimented upon are kept constant.
- There is critical analysis of all data used so that there is no error in their interpretation.
- Employs quantitative or statistical methods—data are transformed into numerical measures and are treated statistically.
- The procedure should be reproducible in nature.

RESEARCH PARADIGMS (FIG. 1.1)

It is the basis belief or worldview or a set of assumptions which directs the researchers to choose the methods of inquiry in fundamental ways. They are:

- Ontological—studies the nature of existence or being as such.
- Epistemological—investigates the origin, nature, methods, and limits of human knowledge.
- Methodological—a set or system of methods, principles, and rules used in any given discipline.
  - Qualitative method
  - Quantitative method
  - Mixed method.

MEANING OF RESEARCH

With the embracing of scientific research, institutes of higher education in the world have been playing a key role in our understanding of humans and issues surrounding them. The main responsibility of academia in the world is to produce and disseminate new knowledge in the society for the well-being of mankind.

Research = New knowledge creation

The new knowledge on a particular topic or area in research is based on rigorous scientific method of collection of data through primary and secondary sources often together with original data collected by means of some research instruments.

Based on the way research question is directed it may be categorized as either **Basic** or **Applied**.

Basic research: It looks at causes, effects, and the nature of things
Applied research: It tries to find answers and solutions to specific problems

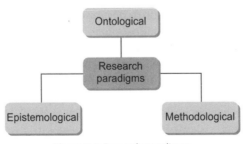

Figure 1.1: Research paradigms.

All research whether basic or applied, focuses on "solving problems" — answering the defined research question(s). Also part of the answering the question is that, research addresses the perceived "problem" of missing or inadequate information on a particular topic. The emphasis and methodology of research may differ between different fields and disciplines, depending on whether it is carried between the Sciences and the Humanities. Thus, Research might be further categorized as follows:

- Research as description
- Research as understanding trends and operations
- Research as explanation.

PHILOSOPHIES OF RESEARCH

Four main categories of research philosophies that guide researcher in the way research is being approached are:

1. Positivist/postpositivist
2. Social constructivist
3. Pragmatic (mixed)
4. Participatory.

The researchers have different views or belief systems which guide them in their research, influencing the decisions they make about how to conduct their studies. The various approaches to research are sometimes called *research paradigms*.

The two main paradigms were the positivist/postpositivist paradigm (quantitative research) and the constructivist paradigm (qualitative research).

Positivist/Postpositivist Paradigm (Quantitative Research)

The positivist attempts to seek "absolute truth" but the postpositivist argument is that this was not appropriate when studying the behavior and actions of people. But, according to "incompatibility theory" which states that the two approaches were irreconcilable due to their very different underlying philosophies. This led to an acceptance that absolute truth can never be found and that research evidence is infallible or not perfect. Generally, Research is an ongoing process, in which data which does not support the theory may result in necessary revisions followed by additional testing. Most of the observable phenomenon can be studied by quantitative research.

Social Constructivist Paradigm

In the social constructivist paradigm, through interaction with other people, the researchers develop subjective understandings and meanings of the experience of the sample studied. Social constructivists believe multiple realities rather than one reality. Based on this theory of reality, researchers are interested to understand the people's experiences and make sense of the world.

Pragmatic Paradigm

The compatibility theory which is contradictory to incompatibility theory acknowledged both the philosophical assumptions but stated that each approach had its strengths and weaknesses and that methods typically used by each could even be mixed in the same study. This is known as the pragmatic paradigm and is generally accepted nowadays as being a valid approach to research.

Participatory Paradigm

A possible fourth paradigm is the advocacy/participatory approach which is often associated with research involving marginalized or vulnerable groups.

QUANTITATIVE RESEARCH (POSITIVIST/POST-POSITIVIST PARADIGM)

Quantitative research is associated with the positivist/postpositivist paradigm. It usually involves measuring, collecting and converting data into numerical form so that statistical calculations can be made through tests and conclusions drawn.

The Process

Normally the research starts with one or more **hypotheses** which are nothing but the questions that includes predictions about possible relationships between the **variables**. In order to find answers to these questions, the researchers will also have various instruments and materials (e.g. paper or computer tests, observation check lists, etc.) and a clearly defined plan of action. Data is collected by various means following a strict procedure and prepared for **statistical analysis**. Nowadays, this is carried out with the aid of sophisticated statistical computer packages (e.g. SPSS, SAS, STRATA, etc.). The analysis enables the researchers to determine whether there is a relationship either could be a simple association or a causal relationship between two or more variables. The results of statistical analyses are presented as statistical significance through **P value**.

Principles (Fig. 1.2)

Objectivity is very important strong point in quantitative research. Positivists believe that only observable experience can be explained and all others are unexplainable. The researchers take great care to avoid any possible bias in the research. Researchers should ensure quality of measurements and control external factors, which might affect the results. The main emphasis of quantitative research is on deductive reasoning, to move from the general to the specific, is also known as a top down approach. The people involved in the study are representative **sample** of the wider population. However, the extent to which generalizations are possible depends to a certain extent on the number of people involved in the study, how and why they were selected. The 'P' stands for probability which is a measure of the likelihood that a particular finding or observed difference is due to chance. The P value is between 0 and 1. The closer the result is to 0, the less likely it is that the observed difference is not due to chance and that there is a real difference between groups. And if the result is closer to 1, the greater the likelihood that the finding is due to chance (random variation) and that there is no difference between the groups. The details of positivist/postpositivist method of research are the main content of this book and are discussed in subsequent chapters.

QUALITATIVE RESEARCH (SOCIAL CONSTRUCTIVIST PARADIGM)

It emphasizes the socially constructed nature of reality
It is about interpreting the significance of human behavior and experiences
It cannot be generalized to other larger groups

The Process

The approach adopted by qualitative researchers tends to be inductive in nature. They develop a theory from the pattern of meaning on the basis of the collected data. This type of specific to the general called a bottom-up approach. Qualitative researchers do not have their predetermined hypotheses with them before the study. The approach to data collection and analysis is methodical but allows for greater

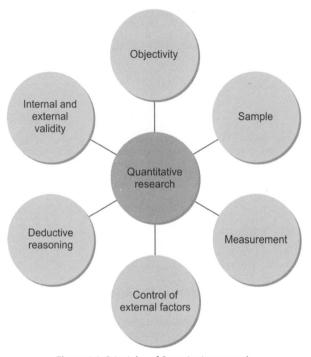

Figure 1.2: Principles of Quantitative research.

flexibility than quantitative research. Data is collected in textual form on the basis of observation and interaction with the participants, e.g. through participant observation, in-depth interviews and focus groups.

Principles (Fig. 1.3)

In qualitative research, researchers use methods which give participants a certain degree of freedom and not forcing them to select from a set of pre-determined responses. This indicates that qualitative research uses a less formal and less rigid approach than that used in quantitative research. As people attribute meaning to their experience it would make no sense to limit the study to the researcher's view of understanding than the experience of the participants. Consequently, the methods used may be more open-ended, less narrow and more exploratory in nature. The researchers are free to go beyond the initial response and ask the participants for their experiences.

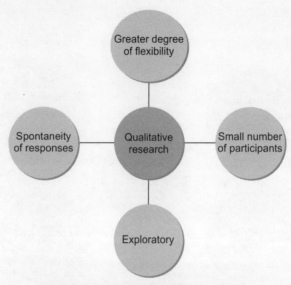

Figure 1.3: Principles of qualitative research.

Qualitative research often involves a smaller number of participants. This may be because the methods used such as in-depth interviews are time and labor intensive but also because a large number of people are not needed for the purposes of statistical analysis or to make generalizations from the results. The smaller number of people and the greater degree of flexibility of qualitative research do not make the study in any way less scientific than a quantitative study involving more subjects and done in rigid manner.

Pragmatic Approach to Research (Mixed Methods)

The pragmatic approach to science involves using the method which appears best suited to the research problem allowing researchers a freedom to use any of the methods, techniques and procedures typically associated with quantitative or qualitative research. They recognize that every method has its own limitations and that using the different approaches for a purpose can be complementary. They may also use different techniques at the same time or one after the other. For example, face-to-face interviews/a focus group discussion to construct a questionnaire to measure attitudes in a large scale sample with the aim of carrying out statistical analysis.

Being able to mix different approaches the pragmatic approach has the advantages of enabling triangulation (a method of validation of data through cross verification from two or more sources).

- Data triangulation—The use of a variety of data sources
- Investigator triangulation—The use of several different researchers
- Theory triangulation—The use of multiple perspectives to interpret the results
- Methodological triangulation—The use of multiple methods to study a research problem

In some studies, qualitative and quantitative methods are used simultaneously. In others, first one approach is used and then the next, with the second part of the study perhaps expanding on the results of the first.

Advocacy/Participatory Approach to Research (Emancipatory)

In this type of research, the researchers adopting an advocacy/ participatory approach feel that the approaches to research such as qualitative, quantitative or mixed methods do not respond to the needs of people from marginalized or vulnerable groups. As this approach aims to bring about positive change in the subjects, this approach is known as emancipatory. As the researchers want their research to directly or indirectly result in some kind of reform, it is important that they try to avoid further marginalizing them. So they may adopt a less neutral position which is usually required in scientific research very much. This might involve interacting informally with the subjects or even living among them (have something in common with the members of the group) and reporting the findings in more personal terms, often using the words of the subjects. Despite criticized for not being objective, this type of research is necessary to understand the thoughts, feelings or behavior of the various members of the group.

RESEARCH METHODS

Figure 1.4 is the concise description of related terminologies of different research paradigms discussed in the previous section.

Experimental Research

The participants of research might be asked to complete various tests and then the results of the groups are compared. This method is the

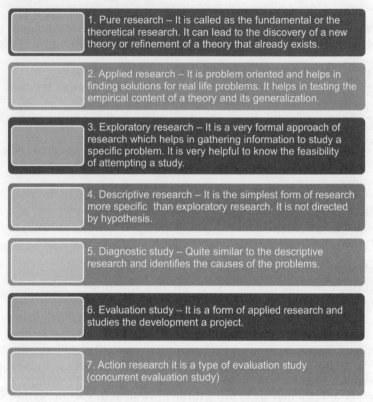

1. Pure research – It is called as the fundamental or the theoretical research. It can lead to the discovery of a new theory or refinement of a theory that already exists.

2. Applied research – It is problem oriented and helps in finding solutions for real life problems. It helps in testing the empirical content of a theory and its generalization.

3. Exploratory research – It is a very formal approach of research which helps in gathering information to study a specific problem. It is very helpful to know the feasibility of attempting a study.

4. Descriptive research – It is the simplest form of research more specific than exploratory research. It is not directed by hypothesis.

5. Diagnostic study – Quite similar to the descriptive research and identifies the causes of the problems.

6. Evaluation study – It is a form of applied research and studies the development a project.

7. Action research it is a type of evaluation study (concurrent evaluation study)

Figure 1.4: Types of research methods.

one to understand causation, effect of intervention or interventions, etc. A study might include an intervention and may use only one group (with in group) sometimes. The researchers might be interested in observing the participants before and after a particular intervention. However, in most cases, there are at least two groups (a between-subjects design) or three groups. One of the groups is known as a **control group** which is not exposed to the intervention. There are various types of research designs in experimental research pre-test, pre-post test design, repeat measures design, factorial design, randomized block design, Solomon four group design. In this type of research the researcher has complete control over the variables. The four elements that the researcher can control are: Manipulation, Control, Random assignment, Random selection.

Survey Method

There are two major types of designs in survey method which are based on the instruments used and span of time the conduct of research involved. Surveys involve collecting information, usually from fairly large groups of people. Based on the instruments used questionnaires, interviews or telephoning are the two major categories of techniques. Based on the time span involved, survey researches are broadly classified into cross-sectional surveys and longitudinal surveys. A brief description about all the various methods are described below.

Questionnaires Method

Questionnaires are a good way to obtain information from a large number of people. They enable people to take their own time, think about it and respond. Participants can state their feelings privately without worrying about the researcher bias. Questionnaires contain multiple choice questions, attitude scales, closed questions and open-ended questions. They usually have a fairly low response rate and incomplete. Questionnaires can be administered in a number of different ways (e.g. sent by post, as email attachments, posted on Internet web sites, handed out personally at door steps). The researchers sometimes may even decide to administer the questionnaire in person which has the advantage of including people who have difficulties in reading and writing (schedules). Before embarking on a survey research using questionnaires, a proper methodology should be followed in developing a questionnaire. The success of this type of research depends on the development of questionnaire which should cover all areas of topic of interest.

Interviews Method

Interviews are usually carried out in person, i.e. face-to-face but can also be administered by telephone or using more advance computer technology. It may be used either as formal or informal approach, letting the interviewee speak freely or by asking specific pre-determined questions to the respondents. A semi-structured approach would enable the interviewee to speak relatively freely and can be helpful for the researchers to have some kind of additional audio or video recording. The types of interviews are face-to-face, phone interview and online interview.

Case Studies Method

Case studies usually involve the detailed study of a particular case. A person-case study or small group-case series. Various methods of data collection and analysis are used but this typically includes observation and interviews and may involve consulting other people and personal or public records.

Observation Method (Participant and Non-participant)

In participant observation method, the researcher becomes part of the group to be observed, and this refers to the emancipatory approach. This enhances gaining the trust of members of the group and able to carry out the observation comfortably. The observations made might be based on what people do, their opinions, explanations, the roles they play, and relationships among them. In non-participant observation methods, the researcher is not part of the group being studied. The researcher realistically and ethically observe the participants of the study.

Observational Trials

Observational trials intended to study the health issues in large groups of people but in natural settings.

Longitudinal studies examine the behavior of a group of people over a fairly lengthy period of time. The group of people involved in this kind of study is known as a **cohort** and they share a certain characteristic within a defined period. If the researcher is following a group of people from a specific point in time onwards, working forward is known as prospective approach and working backwards is known as retrospective approach. This retrospective approach is not always a reliable method and may be problematic as some people may forget, exaggerate or idealize their behavior. For this reason, a prospective study is generally attempted depending on the research question.

Cross-sectional studies examine the behavior of a group of people at a specific point in time and help to remove assumptions. The data gathered from participants with varied characteristics and demographics are known as variables.

FURTHER READING

1. Introduction to Research in the Health Sciences E-Book Stephen Polgar, Shane A. Thomas Elsevier Health Sciences, 24-Oct-2011 - Medical - 344 pages.
2. Introduction to Research Methods: A practical guide for anyone undertaking a research project Catherine Dawson Hachette UK, 29-May-2009 - Science - 160 pages.
3. Introduction to Research in Education Donald Ary, Lucy Cheser Jacobs, Christine K. Sorensen Irvine, David Walker Cengage Learning, 01-Jan-2013 - Business & Economics - 720 pages.

Research in Physiotherapy

RESEARCH

The word "Research" many a times causes fear and panic among students as a bitter taste subject until he or she gets well-versed with the process involved in it. Research is not something that is out of bound from our life. With a wide range of information and knowledge glut on every sphere of life, there is a need to channelize ourselves to find the right kind of information at the right time to lead into a solution for the question we have in our mind. We, in our everyday life keep doing research in many works that we are engaged with. Be it a travel plan, or purchasing a book, selecting a course for a career and so on. We keep asking in our mind. "Which is the best book for a specific subject?" or "Which is the best course to study?" Then we set out on a research process by searching for relevant information asking people associated with our search, various sources like books, internet, etc., until we come to a conclusion. Similarly the advent and advancement of various things that we see in the area of health world around us can be attributed to this process of systematic search towards a better understanding of us.

The research process consists of a series of steps in an orderly manner linking information towards the rightful knowledge to lead into a chain of interlinking knowledge. These steps that are followed are similar in any area of research. The process starts by development of a research question in an already existing piece of information and moves on by exploring the relationship between the developed question, the methodological process undertaken, information gained from the process as data and finally analysing the processed information. However, the methodological process used in various situations, type of data that are collected in various types of research process and analysis of the data vary which form the different types of research. The purpose of this book is to give an insight into the details of various process used in different situations in research methodology in a simple manner. Thus research forms an integral part of human understanding of the world to the universe we live in and is a constant on-going process. Research has been defined in various ways by various authors. We have attempted in this book to simplify this process of scientific enquiry where students go confusing by relating to them examples from health sciences which they frequently come across in their professional life.

Definitions

Research has been defined in a number of different ways. The following are the few definitions:

"In the broadest sense of the word, the definition of research includes any gathering of data, information and facts for the advancement of knowledge". — *Martyn Shuttleworth*

"Research is a process of steps used to collect and analyze information to increase our understanding of a topic or issue".
— *Creswell*

"It is a systematic study of trend or event which involves careful collection, presentation, analysis and interpretation of quantitative data or facts that relates man's thinking with reality".
— *Jeff L Homeres*

"A systematic investigation, including research development, testing and evaluation, designed to develop or contribute to generalizable knowledge."

Webster Dictionary defines research in more detail as *"a studious inquiry or examination."*

"Research is the manipulation of things, concepts or symbols for the purpose of generalizing to extend, correct or verify knowledge, whether the knowledge aids construction of theory or in practice of an art." — *Encyclopedia of Social Sciences*

Characteristics of Research

- Research is logical and objective. It focuses on search for knowledge.
- Research is Empirical, Systematic and is based on scientific method.

- It is cyclical in nature—starts with a problem and ends with a problem.
- It finds out relationship between two or more variables.
- All variables are controlled except those that are experimented upon are kept constant.
- There is critical analysis of all data used so that there is no error in their interpretation.
- Employs quantitative or statistical methods—data are transformed into numerical measures and are treated statistically.
- Research is conducted in a methodical manner without bias using systematic method and procedures.
- Research designs and procedures are repeated to enable researcher to arrive at valid and conclusive results.

HISTORY OF RESEARCH

The word research is derived from the middle period French word "recherche", which means "to go about seeking". The earliest recorded use of the term was in 1577. Research is the process continuum of finding solution for the raised question - a scientific and systematic search for pertinent information on a specific topic. It is considered to be formal, systematic, intensive process of carrying out the scientific method of analysis, resulting in some conclusions. That way research can be termed as an art of doing scientific investigation and can be said as an on-going process of continuum since time immemorial. Hence, it is not a new phenomenon and can be said as has been happening since human evolution.

PRINCIPLES OF RESEARCH

1. *Objectivity*: The objective of research work needs to be clearly described and common precept be used.
2. *Use of scientific process*: The research process used must be explained in detail allowing other researchers to repeat the research in a systematic way.
3. *Planning*: The design needs to be prepared in a most scientific way and all aspects of resources, time period, constraints and procedural factors be considered.
4. *Continuity*: The study has to be conducted in a way that principle of continuity is guaranteed. Validate existing theories or generate new ones.

5. *Integrity*: The researcher must document with complete frankness, weaknesses in procedural design and assess their impact on the results.

6. *Reliability*: The validity and reliability of data needs to be examined with care.

7. *Adequacy of data*: The analysis of data must be sufficient to disclose its significance and the approaches to analysis employed must be suitable.

8. *Structure*: This would mean that research is organized with particular sequence as per the well-defined set of rules. Guessing and intuition in arriving at conclusions are discarded.

9. *Logic*: What this means is that research is well guided by the rules of logical reasoning and logical process of induction and deduction are used.

10. *Empiricism*: This means that research is connected basically to one or more facets of a real situation and deals with concrete data which gives a basis for external validity of research outcomes.

11. *Replicability*: This principle enables research outcome to be validated by replicating the research and thus creating a sound basis for decision.

12. *Economics*: Research must be completed within the allotted financial resources

13. *Time frame*: Frame research needs to be finished in the established time frame.

GOALS AND PURPOSES OF RESEARCH

Three important goals for which research is carried out are Descriptive, Explanatory and Predictive and are briefly explained below.

Descriptions allow us to establish generalizations and universals from the findings of the research. For example, information gathered by research on a large population informs us about the characteristics of the population on the topic in question and helps us able to describe as to how variable react for a group or single person. Description from a previous research helps us to plan, decide, prepare and act based on the results attained from the previous research.

One of the most important goal and purpose of the research is **explanation**. This refers to the cause or causes of the phenomenon. The main explanatory factors to understand the causative effect of a phenomenon are covariation of events, proper time-order sequence, elimination of plausible causes.

- To understand the relationship between two variables, methodologies and tests are used to measure and test the existence and strength of relationships which is called covariance of events.
- Another explanation of the causation of research is time-order sequence. For example, 1 to cause 2, 1 must precede 2.
- Another explanation of causation is elimination of non-binders which are controlled. For example, when A is the reason for existence of B, C should be controlled.

Prediction is another important goal and purpose of research. Predictions sometimes made in the form of hypotheses, concerning the relationship between or among variables. Hypotheses are derived from theories, or interrelated sets of concepts that explain a body of data and make predictions. Also, predictions are made with varying degrees of certainty.

PHYSIOTHERAPY FIELD

Physiotherapy is a profession by definition encourages the physiotherapists to practice their therapeutic techniques based on strong available evidence. It can be said confidently that the evolution of the profession of Physiotherapy has been based on the systematic basis of scientific research, and as such roles of Physiotherapists are getting better defined with more and more research in the medical research. The roles of physiotherapists in major areas of health are also well-defined and with scientific reasoning of concepts used, following are the few definitions and role description of physiotherapists internationally and in India:

"Physiotherapists assess, plan and implement rehabilitative programs that improve or restore human motor functions, maximize movement ability, relieve pain syndromes, and treat or prevent physical challenges associated with injuries, diseases and other impairments. They apply a broad range of physical therapies and techniques such as movement, ultrasound, heating, laser and other techniques. They may develop and implement programmes for screening and prevention of common physical ailments and disorders".(WHO)(ISCO-2264)

"Physical therapy is a dynamic profession with an established theoretical and scientific base and widespread clinical applications in the restoration, maintenance, and promotion of optimal physical function. Physical therapists are health care professionals who help individuals maintain, restore, and improve movement, activity, and

functioning, thereby enabling optimal performance and enhancing health, well-being, and quality of life. Their services prevent, minimize, or eliminate impairments of body functions and structures, activity limitations, and participation restrictions".(APTA)

"Physical therapy provides services to individuals and populations to develop, maintain and restore maximum movement and functional ability throughout the lifespan. This includes providing services in circumstances where movement and function are threatened by ageing, injury, pain, diseases, disorders, conditions or environmental factors. Functional movement is central to what it means to be healthy. Physical therapy is concerned with identifying and maximising quality of life and movement potential within the spheres of promotion, prevention, treatment/intervention, habilitation and rehabilitation. This encompasses physical, psychological, emotional, and social wellbeing. Physical therapy involves the interaction between the physical therapist, and patients/clients, other health professionals, families, care givers and communities in a process where movement potential is assessed and goals are agreed upon, using knowledge and skills unique to physical therapists." (WCPT)

"As per Delhi State Physiotherapy Council Act "Physiotherapy" means physiotherapeutic system of medicine which includes examination, treatment, advice and instructions to any person preparatory to or for the purpose of or in connection with movement dysfunction, bodily malfunction, physical disorder, disability, healing and pain from trauma and disease, physical and mental conditions using physical agents including exercise, mobilization, manipulation, mechanical and electrotherapy, activity and devices or diagnosis, treatment and prevention". (Reference: http://delhiassembly.nic.in/ aspfile/billspassed/141997.htm)

"As per Maharashtra State OTPT Council Act: "Physiotherapy" means a branch of modern medical science which includes examination, assessment, interpretation, physical diagnosis, planning and execution of treatment and advice to any person for the purpose of preventing, correcting, alleviating and limiting dysfunction, acute and chronic bodily malfunction including life saving measures via chest physiotherapy in the intensive care units, curing physical disorders or disability, promoting physical fitness, facilitating healing and pain relief and treatment of physical and psychosomatic disorders through modulating physiological and physical response using

physical agents, activities and devices including exercise, mobilization, manipulations, therapeutic ultrasound, electrical and thermal agents and electrotherapy for diagnosis, treatment and prevention". (Reference: http://www.msotptcouncil.com/OTPTActs.aspx).

"As per Tamil Nadu State Physiotherapy Council Government Order "Physiotherapy" means health care profession which includes examination, treatment, advice and instructions to any person preparatory to or for the purpose of or in connection with movement dysfunction, bodily malfunction, physical disorder, disability, healing and pain from trauma and disease, physical and mental conditions using physical agents including exercise, mobilization, manipulation, mechanical and electrotherapy, activity and devices or diagnosis, treatment and prevention". (Ref: G.O. (Ms) No.338 Health and Family Welfare Department, Dated 16.10.2008, with Amendments G.O (Ms) No.281 Dated 09-09-2009, of Health and Family Welfare (Z1) Department).

"As per Gujarat State Physiotherapy Council Act "Physiotherapy" means a branch of modern medical science which includes examination, assessment, interpretation, physical diagnosis, planning and execution of treatment and advice to any person for the purpose of preventing, correcting, alleviating and limiting dysfunction, acute and chronic bodily malfunction, including life saving measures via chest physiotherapy in the intensive care units curing physical disorders and disabilities, curing physical disorders or disability, promoting physical fitness, facilitating healing and pain relief and treatment of physical and psychosomatic disorders through modulating physiological and physical response using physical agents, activities and devices including exercises, mobilization, manipulations, mechanical, electrical and thermal agents and electrotherapy including therapeutic ultrasound, therapeutic laser, electrotherapy including electrophysiology for diagnosis, treatment and prevention".

"As per Government of India Quality Council of India, Survey Report and Recommendations of Clinical Establishments – Page-11 Physiotherapy Definition: The treatment of disease, bodily defects, or bodily weaknesses by physical remedies, as massage, special exercises, etc., rather than by drugs". (Reference:http://clinicalestablishments.nic. in/WriteReadData/384).

One of the reason why research should be carried out in Physio-therapy is that the most definitions above describing the role of Physiotherapists in different places is a typical example that variation in practice is existent. If only the role play a profession becomes uniform will it become easy for practising professional to provide efficient and effective care? A lifelong learning in the pursuit of in depth knowledge is central to research in Physiotherapy. Hence, clinical research is becoming an integral part of routine practice worldwide.

RESEARCH IN PHYSIOTHERAPY

Clinical research in Physiotherapy is as important to the profession as any other medical field. As mentioned previously, the profession of Physiotherapy development is based on a strong foundation of scientific research. The profession grew alongside through times when research in science was making strides in the understanding of the universe and still a long way to go in the exploration of what it can offer to health of a human being. Research in Physiotherapy has become integral part of academic curricula from undergraduate level. Reviews suggest that there is more evidence to suggest that there is a uniformity of research being a main part of Physiotherapy academic curricula throughout the world. This would help in defining the roles of Physiotherapists and more importantly benefits to the patients in the form of better health care.

Increasingly physiotherapy research is being carried out in India in increasing numbers over the years. Research in physiotherapy field in India is an important part in the curriculum towards the gaining of a postgraduate degree or Doctorate (masters or PhD in physiotherapy) in universities or affiliated colleges which is helping in the expanding of the knowledge base in physiotherapy. An individual or independent research is rare due to circumstantial limitations. Predominantly Physiotherapeutic researches in India that are carried out are on quantitative research. Many a time, research scholars adopt a pre-post study design with two or more groups and more than two times measurements of outcome measures. This scenario leads to application of statistical tests like parametric/non-parametric or Anova based on assumptions and study design. A statistical significance of 'p' value less than 0.05 is considered as difference existing between the groups on outcome measures, leading to a conclusion that the alternative hypothesis is accepted as a positive result or evidence for clinical practice. Hence, there is a large gap in the way research is to be informed to the student and clinical population based on the kind of information on research methodology. Therefore we felt there is a need for a kind of book which inform about the research in a simpler language. This may promote interest in better quality researches and addition to the knowledge base primarily focussing our attention on Physiotherapy and Allied Health, why not, if can also serve to a wider extent to other branches of health sciences. Engagement in high quality research would lead to better evidence base for an effective practice.

EVIDENCE

The available body of facts or information indicating whether a belief or proposition is true or valid. — Oxford Dictionary

Evidence is anything that you see, experience, read, or are told that causes you to believe that something is true or has really happened. — Collins Dictionary

Sackett et al, described evidence as, "The conscientious, explicit and judicious use of current best evidence in making decisions about the care of an individual".

Development of every piece of information in a research conducted with appropriate manipulation of variables to understand the real outcome, experience of a phenomenon in an unbiased manner forms an effective piece of information in the knowledge base as evidence. This evidence development is the need to stick the piece of information at the right time to be a solution to the problem.

In medicine, Evidence based practice is a mean of integrating individual clinical expertise with the best available external clinical evidence from systematic search. As described by Sackett (1997), "By best available external clinical evidence we mean clinically relevant research, often from the basic sciences of medicine, but especially from patient centered clinical research into the accuracy and precision of diagnostic tests including the clinical examination, the power of prognostic markers, and the efficacy and safety of therapeutic, rehabilitative, and preventive regimens." Without current best external evidence, practice risks becoming rapidly out of date, to the detriment of patients. Good clinicians use both individual clinical expertise and the best available external evidence, and neither alone is enough. The information that is generated are categorized based on authenticity with which the research is performed and form the levels of evidence.

ROLE OF EVIDENCE IN THE CURRENT PRACTICE OF PHYSIOTHERAPY

"Physical therapy profession recognizes the use of evidence based practice as central to providing high quality care and decreasing variation in practice – APTA, 2017. Given the development of physiotherapy from a profession into an autonomous profession in the end of last century in areas where scientific medicine is practised aggressively, it can be said that this development owes a lot to the research knowledge deciphered from various levels. This research knowledge is and has been effective as an evidence base for betterment in physiotherapy practice. However uniformity in practice is far from actual due to the variation in the understanding of Evidence-Based Practice (EBP), dissemination of research information. As more and more research is being undertaken the scientific understanding of a process is getting better established, and it becomes imperative that research needs to be carried out keeping this building block of evidence as base. EBP becomes very important for the profession of Physiotherapy as the profession deal with patients' decision. One of the corner stone of EBP is the informed choices of patients, as the part of physiotherapy in the current medical practice is very much patient centered, the role of EBP becomes very imperative for the practice of the Physiotherapy profession.

The rigorous search of evidence data bases regarding the quality and applicability of physiotherapy assessment and treatment principles could be an eye opener for the regular clinical practicing clinician. The present search and conclusions of studies produced an ambiguous speculation of current practice. So further in depth research work is necessary to justify and validate the current practice. Here the readers are requested to access the evidences in appropriate databases whenever it is necessary. Hence it is not using of evidence base alone, but critical appraisal of evidence is very much central to the practice of physiotherapy so that the practicing clinician leads into the right kind of information at the right time for effective delivery of service. It is expected that this skill in the appraisal is an important part to avoid variation in practice which would eventually lead to providing of better and effective care. Hence the role of EBP is and will remain central for better care in the years to come in the practice of Physiotherapy.

FURTHER READING

1. Condon C, et al. Ability of physiotherapists to undertake evidence-based practice steps: a scoping review. Physiotherapy 2016;102(1): 10-19.
2. Mota da Silva T, et al. What do physical therapists think about evidence-based practice? A systematic review. Manual Therapy 2015;20(3): 388-40.
3. Scurlock-Evans L, et al. Evidence-based practice in physiotherapy: a systematic review of barriers, enablers and interventions. Physiotherapy 2014;100(3): 208-19.

Research Process

RESEARCH PROCESS

Physiotherapy profession has made huge strides over the past few decades and it is not without rigorous research that the importance of physiotherapy in health care has been established and continued growth in research information is essential further for betterment in healthcare. The way to collect this information through a scientific manner is known as research. Scientific research process is a systematic, logical, empirical and replicable vigorous impersonal mode of procedure required by the demand of the scientific enquiry. It may include various steps not following any specific order. If a researcher is intended to find the truth, then he/she must have information which is gathered by means of collecting data. However collection of data is a complex and difficult process. In short, research process is the way to conceptualize, plan, conduct a research study and communicating **(Writing up the study)** the results to the audience. Thus, research process could be understood as one of the on-going process of planning, searching, discovery, reflection, synthesis, revision, and learning as shown in Bruce's reflective model **(Fig. 3.1)**. The following five phases outline a simple and effective strategy for conducting effective research:

I. The conceptual phase: The process of developing refining abstract ideas
- Identifying the research question
- Reviewing the related and relevant literature
- Refining the research question

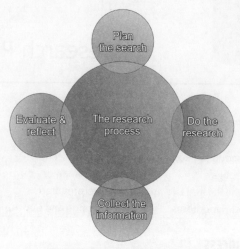

Figure 3.1: The research process.

Activities by the researcher—creative thinking, rethinking, insightful theory making, making decision and reviewing ideas by discussion.

II. Phase of construction of research design

- Developing the study design: Identification of variables, construction of operational definitions for variables
- Identifying the population and sample-selection, inclusion and exclusion criteria, randomization and allocation
- Identify the data collection methods–protocls/procedures, and tools
- Access and ethical issues of the study
- Carrying out a pilot study before the main research.

III. Empiric phase: Measurements

- Recruiting participants
- Collecting data—timing of data collection, duration of data collection and quality of data collection
- Preparing the data—data control, data coding.

IV. Analytic phase

- Data analysis—examine for completeness and accuracy of data, systemic processing of data, classification of data, using statistical methods
- Drawing conclusion—interpretation and making sense of the results.

V. Disseminative phase—communicating the results to the audience as a journal publication or presenting it in a large gathering such as conferences at various levels.

STEPS IN CONDUCTING RESEARCH (RESEARCH PROCESS) (FIG. 3.2)

The phases of research are grouped based on the activities that are related in the research process, and divided distinctively based on the action that is carried out into steps for further understanding. The various steps in the process of research which a researcher should follow during the conduct of research is mentioned below. Though

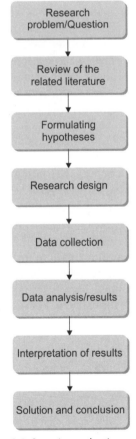

Figure 3.2: Steps in conducting research.

the steps are series in nature there may be overlap of the steps along with forward and backward feedback influence of one on another.

RESEARCH PROBLEM (FIG. 3.3)

"A problem is an interrogative sentence or statement that asks what relation exists between two or more variable". — **Kerlinger 1956**

The researchers can formulate the research problem on a topic of their interest or as the result outcome of their clinical practice. The researcher may refine the problem after following many steps starting from selecting the area, finding the source, narrowing and evaluating, framing the statement and formatting it to make it researchable as well as feasible. The words and vocabulary in the statement should reflect for a normal person the underlying intend behind the search of knowledge for which the supposed research is being undertaken. However, there may be minimal altercations in the words that may be allowed without sacrificing the original intend of the problem for which this research is planned. There are two types of research problems; one states the nature (descriptive) and the other one relationship between the variables of interest.

REVIEW OF THE RELATED LITERATURE

"Review of literature is a process of finding the sources of relevant material for particular topic or subject." — **Galvan 2005**

From deciding the statement of the research problem, the next step in the process is to know the current level of knowledge base in the topic of interest. This will lead to whether our research question and the conduct of research is tuned to further add the knowledge base. This needs a rigorous search for the related literature through various knowledge resources called as literature review. The literature review is the eye opener for carrying out research. It includes facts,

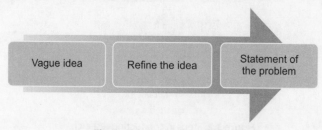

Figure 3.3: Research problem.

concepts and previous research findings from academic journals, reports, books, conference proceedings and published or unpublished theses. A vigorous search is very necessary to find out the information related to the research from the sources. The researcher may end up collecting a range of different documents such as papers reporting original research, reviews, editorials, methodological papers, policy documents and guidelines. A flowchart on the steps that are usually the components of literature review is mentioned below **(Fig. 3.4)**. Also, the steps to be followed in internet search during conducting a literature review is available through various internet sites or a contact with most of the librarian in academic centers would be useful. A comprehensive and thorough scrutiny for latest knowledge on the topic of interest through literature review would be effective for research to be beneficial in its purpose.

FORMULATING HYPOTHESES

"Hypothesis is a formal statement that presents the expected relationship between an independent and dependent variable."
— Creswell, 1994

From the collected unbiased knowledge through the literature review, framing of hypothesis is the next step in the conduct of research. The hypothesis should be based on the prediction that the researcher arrive at based on the premise that he develop from the

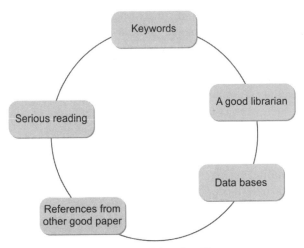

Figure 3.4: Review of the related literature.

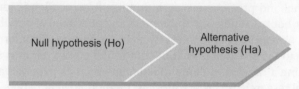

Figure 3.5: Hypothesis.

literature review. A hypothesis is a tentative solution to the problem of interest for the researcher (Shrewd guess or inference, an assumption or proposition, temporary statement or probable outcome). The hypothesis should be simple, clear, precise and reasonable. Moreover it should be purposeful and testable. There are two types of hypothesis (Fig. 3.5):

- Null hypothesis (Ho)—a negative statement
- Alternative hypothesis (Ha)—a positive statement
  Hypothesis serves as a guiding light in the world of darkness and decides the direction of the research work. Design of the experiment is revolve around the hypothesis, hence it is important for the hypothesis to be on the intended aim of the research.

RESEARCH DESIGN

"Research design is a planned sequence of the entire process involved in the conducting of as research study". — **Miller 2002**

The type of design is going to be driven by the nature of research question. The methodological choices that a researcher is opted with are: taking a predominantly quantitative approach; taking a predominantly qualitative approach; or taking an approach that draws on both quantitative and qualitative methodologies (mixed methods). Whatever the methodological design that is chosen, a research design is the arrangement of conditions for collection and analysis of data. On that basis, designs are classified into:

1. Sampling design
2. Observational design
3. Operational design
4. Statistical design.

A good research design should be free from bias, eliminate confounding of variables and control of extraneous variables and should measure what the research question is purported to measure. The important characteristics of the research design are objectivity,

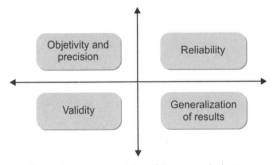

Figure 3.6: Characteristics of the research design.

reliability and validity of the methods and generalization of results to the society (Fig. 3.6).

DATA COLLECTION (FIG. 3.7)

"Data collection is the process of gathering and measuring information on variables of interest, in an established systematic fashion that enables one to answer stated research questions, test hypotheses, and evaluate outcomes".   **— Unknown**

Data collection is the most exciting or enjoyable part of the research process for most of the researchers. It requires more patience and serious involvement as it may extent for weeks, months, maybe even years. The collection of appropriate and adequate data for the research study is essential for deriving empirical evidence as conclusion. Tools or instruments such as questionnaires, checklist, inventories, rating scales, interviews and observations are used for data collection. The data can be primary or secondary. For example, in a cross-sectional study with an aim to know the amount of different types of fishes caught in the month of August in a lake near your locality. In a quantitative study like this the data collected will be in numbers, but the based on the amount of fish that are caught the way you calculate the data would be in kilograms or in individual numbers. But the data that is collected by the researcher is the most essential part of the study that we conduct which may provide valuable information and help us in decision making in time. In short it is the ground work based on which the whole study revolves and there are number of ways through which we can analyze the data which is the next stage of the process. Similarly, as mentioned before based on the

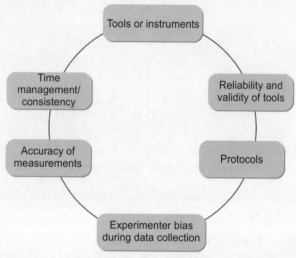

Figure 3.7: Data collection.

type of research, in a qualitative research, the type of collected data is different and most of the time will not be in numbers.

DATA ANALYSIS

"Various analytic procedures provide a way of drawing inductive inferences from data and distinguishing the signal (the phenomenon of interest) from the noise (statistical fluctuations) present in the data". — **Shamoo and Resnik 2003**

It is the process of testing the hypotheses through various statistical tests or otherwise is the process of systematically applying statistical and logical techniques to describe, illustrate, condense and evaluate data. Parametric tests, non-parametric tests, correlational and regression analyses could be used. The collected data should be checked and cleaned before applying the tests. Data analysis includes coding operation, tabulation, appropriate statistical formulae and hypothesis testing for significance as various steps (Fig. 3.8).

INTERPRETATION

It is nothing but interpreting and understanding the derived results of the present study in line with the previous research study findings, theory and hypotheses to know whether they support or contradict the present research study outcome to generalize the results. For

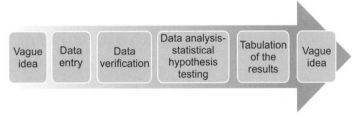

Figure 3.8: Data analysis.

qualitative research, data analysis will involve identifying common pattern in responses and analyzing them in reaching research aims and objectives. In case of quantitative research, it involves critical analysis and interpretation of figures and numbers, to find the rationale behind the development of new findings. Thus, whatever the type of research, data analysis gives the much needed comparison with the primary findings from the literature review and to understand relationship through the new knowledge evolved through the research in the understanding towards reality for which the supposed research is undertaken.

SOLUTION AND CONCLUSION

The findings from the research form basis for inference on the topic of interest which may be solution for a problem or new dimension in the knowledge base. Thus, Solutions are the findings which are derived as statements of factual information based on sorting/coding in case of qualitative research and statistical analysis of data in case of quantitative research. The interpretation of the findings which could be generalized is known as conclusion or solution of the problem.

FURTHER READING

1. Bouma GD, Ling R. The research process. Oxford University Press, USA, 2004.
2. Bordens KS, Abbott BB. Research design and methods: A process approach, 5th ed. New York: McGraw-Hill, 2002.
3. Fox DJ. The Research Process in Education. New York: Holt, Rinehart and Winston, 1969.

Research Problem and Literature Review

RESEARCH PROBLEM

A research problem, in general, refers to some difficulty which researchers experience in the context of either a theoretical or practical situation or wants to obtain a solution for the same.

A **research problem** is a statement about an area of concern. The selection of a problem is governed by reflective thinking (convergent, divergent, reflective and scientific thinking). In reflective thinking individual conceived a new solution for an old problem. An identified research problem needs to be framed into appropriate worded statement.

CHARACTERISTICS OF A PROBLEM

Before defining a problem, it is essential to understand what constitutes a problem. Figure 4.1 mentions four distinctive ways that a given statement can be considered a problem.

NECESSITY OF DEFINING THE PROBLEM

It is very important that the researcher define a problem for the following reasons:

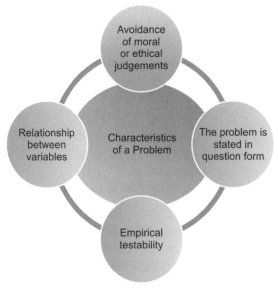

Figure 4.1: Characteristics of a problem.

- To avoid deviating from the goal, the definition of a problem sets the direction of the study
- To derive the objectives the study
- Proper selection of methodology for the study
- Selection of variables for the study
- Clarity for the readers about what is going to be discussed in the study article
- The definition helps the researcher to control subjectivity or biases of the researcher
- Makes the study feasible.

STATEMENT OF RESEARCH PROBLEM

Statement is a clear and concise written description of the issue. Normally the statement is one or two sentences in length which briefly outlines the problem addressed by the study.

A good **problem statement/Research-worthy problem statement** should address all six questions: what, how, where, when, why, and who.

CRITERIA FOR THE SELECTION OF THE PROBLEM SUGGESTED BY GOOD AND SCATES

Good and Scates defined following criteria for a specific issue to be considered as a problem.

- Novelty and avoidance of unnecessary duplications
- Importance for the field represented and implementation
- Interest, intellectual curiosity, and drive
- Training and personal qualifications
- Availability of data and method
- Special equipment and working conditions
- Approachability of the sample
- Sponsorship and administrative cooperation
- Hazards, penalties and handicaps
- Cost and returns
- Time factor.

STATEMENT OF PURPOSE AND OBJECTIVES OF RESEARCH PROBLEM

Once it is identified that the research problem is a gap in the knowledge, to satisfy the main criteria mentioned above, a statement of purpose on it would give an idea of expanding it further exploration. Statement of the problem should contain three components (Fig. 4.2):

1. It should state the given background of the problem.
2. The new assumption of the researcher in that area of research.
3. The intention (objective) of the researcher in the current research.

Example:

Excess body weight is related to significant morbidity and mortality among the people. However, less is known about the relationship of body weight to health-related quality of life (HRQOL), especially for

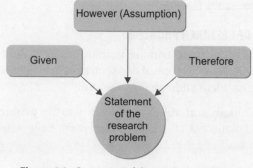

Figure 4.2: Statement of the research problem.

Indian populations. In the statement above, the given problem is there any relationship between excess body weight and HRQOL. Therefore, the aim of the study was to find out the relationship of excess weight and HRQOL in a general population sample from Surat, Gujarat.

The new assumption may be, from the researcher's experience and his knowledge search, that there is no relationship or some other factors may be responsible apart from excess bodyweight. This is the second step in the statement of the problem.

Thirdly, the ways and means by which the researcher intends to carry out the research forms the third statement of the problem. This represents the objective the researcher intends to find by addressing the problem.

In any narration, presentation of statement in the right way is very important. Kerlinger has identified three criteria of good Problem Statements.

1. A problem should be concerned with relation between two or more variables.
2. It should be stated "clearly and unambiguously in question form".
3. It should be amenable to empirical testing.

PROBLEM STATEMENT MODELS

This is the underlying principle on which any problem statement is based on. Any problem statement can be zeroed into the below mentioned three models. As it is not the purpose of this book to explain in detail about the statement only three models are mentioned below.

1. Action-knowledge conflict model.
2. Knowledge-knowledge conflict model.
3. Policy-Action conflict (knowledge void) model.

THEORETICAL FRAMEWORK OF THE PROBLEM (FORM OF PROBLEM)

These are ways in which the researcher can view the direction that the problem can be taken.

If it is applied to the above mentioned example for problem statement, then, one way of looking at it is "body weight and mortality are related" in one kind of population. Similarly the same can be applied so many different populations. Also another theory that can be formed is "if there are any other factors that are related to morbidity and mortality apart from excess weight. Thus theory of a problem can be developed in two fundamental ways.

Extending a previous work by studying new populations in new setting and in different cultural and socioeconomic group	Extending a previous work by adding new variables

MERITS OF DESCRIBING A RESEARCH PROBLEM

Merits of a research problem give an insight into the direction of the research that the researcher is undertaking and align the real understanding to the statement of purpose. The below mentioned guide may be useful for the researcher to make valuable conclusion regarding the research that he/she is undertaking. Hildreth Hoke McAshan has proposed an objective guide for judging the merits of a problem. They are:

- Is the problem really important for the field of research?
- Is the problem interesting to the other people of the field?
- Is the problem a real and concurrent one? And display originality and creativeness?
- Does the researcher really concerned with finding the solution?
- Does the researcher able to state hypotheses from the problem in a testable form?
- Will the researcher learn something new from this problem?
- Does the researcher understand the relationship of this specific problem to the broader problem area?
- Does the researcher able to generalize results to some population?
- Will some other intelligent person be able to replicate the study?
- Is there any practical application of results?

REVIEW OF LITERATURE

Review of literature is a step in every learning curve, in which we look back into the evidences on the knowledge on a particular topic. The author or person interested to know information on a particular topic go back and forth in time to retrieve, assess, analyze the knowledge that has been gained on the topic of interest and has led to the current level. Hence reviewing is an essential step in bridging knowledge gap and new dimension in our understanding of a particular thing. The following are the objectives, features and intended outcomes of the review of literature.

- The studies found in the literature related to selected area

- The review should describe, summarize, evaluate and clarify this literature
- Theoretical basis for the research
- The framework for topic/subject area. It defines key terms, definitions and terminology
- The main types of literature reviews are: *evaluative, exploratory*, and *instrumental*
- A careful literature review is usually 15 to 30 pages and could be longer.

PURPOSE OF REVIEW OF LITERATURE

The purpose of literature review is to explain and inform the process, its findings and what can be done on the issue of interest. The following bullet points describe about the experiences that a person undergo, understand and the benefit of doing a literature review—in other words the purpose of doing a literature review.

- Explaining to the reader what the problem is that you're tackling
- Explaining which approaches have been tried before
- Explaining why they failed (otherwise it would be solved and no longer a problem)
- Explaining what your approach will be
- Explaining the background to your approach (previous work, etc.)
- Provide a context for the research
- Justify the research
- Ensure the research hasn't been done before (or that it is not just a "replication study")
- Show where the research fits into the existing body of knowledge
- Enable the researcher to learn from previous theory on the subject
- Illustrate how the subject has been studied previously
- Highlight flaws in previous research
- Outline gaps in previous research
- Show that the work is adding to the understanding and knowledge of the field
- Help refine, refocus or even change the topic.

THE PROCESS OF REVIEW OF LITERATURE (WHAT YOU SEARCH; WHAT YOU SEARCH IT FOR; HOW YOU SEARCH IT)

The process of reviewing the literature requires different kinds of cognitive activities and ways of thinking from the researcher. The higher functions that are involved are generally listed below while doing a review.

Benjamin Bloom's revised taxonomy of the cognitive domain (ways of thinking)
- Remembering
- Understanding
- Applying
- Analysing
- Evaluating
- Creating

SOURCES OF REVIEW OF LITERATURE

Literature review doesn't limit itself to the current sources of knowledge base such as internet and its contents. Rather review can trace as far back as possible to the written literatures and evidences in any form related to topic of interest. However, as far as scientific knowledge is concerned, the existing information can mostly be traced to written and internet sources. Table 4.1 Below mentions the list of internet sources which provide information on various subjects and commonly used for literature review. The development of computer, World Wide Web or online database has enabled the review of literature much easier and comprehensive with proper search strategy. Otherwise the search for knowledge was mostly hand search which used to be cumbersome as the many times it used to be limited in the resources that are traced as the search strategy could not be widened due to physical limitations. A short description on search strategy is mentioned in the subsequent sections.

Table 4.1: Sources of review of literature

Sources	Used in
Medline, science direct, Biomed central	Medicine
Embase	Biomedical and pharmacology
CINAHL	Nursing and allied health
Psych INFO	Psychology
ERIC	Education related
Pedro	Physiotherapy related
World cat database. WWW.worldlib.com www.Qspace.library.queensu.ca www.inflibnet.ac.in, www.vidhyanidhi.org.in, www.mgutheses.in, www.sodhganga.in, www.openthesis.org.	For dissertations, theses and abstracts

Contd...

Contd...

Sources	Used in
Archives of physical medicine and rehabilitation	For conference publications
Index of scientific and technical proceedings (ISTP)	For published contents in conferences ·

STRATEGIES FOR REVIEW OF LITERATURE

As mentioned above the search strategy has to be as wider as possible to collate the best of knowledge to make us reach to the reality of the current problem that we have chosen to study. Algorithm of search strategy for internet related sources can be found in internet. For example, Google, Youtube offers a wide range of advices on how to do literature search in a practical manner so that relevant sources are not missed or left out.

Strategies for review of literature (Kirby S, Greaves L, Reid C 2006):

- Start with handbooks, overviews and review their references
- Track the authors and their works
- Use library guides
- Record the key words and their contexts
- Establish a personal search pattern (Data bases, types of materials, track strategy, etc.)
- Narrowing of searches and finding key authors
- Use citation indexes and manage references.

PRINCIPLES OF WRITING LITERATURE REVIEW

Literature review can be written as a part of a Research paper, Proposal, Thesis or Dissertation, to learn the topic, to improve understanding of the topic, to develop new ideas, to demonstrate the researcher's knowledge about the topic.

Starting the Write up of Literature Review

- Find a relevant research question. And make the statement of the research question as specific as possible.
- Search for articles and books which are related to the context of the research using the library or an online database (http://scholar.google.com.tr/) to find general reference tools, primary and secondary sources. General reference tools guide us to where

to look to locate other sources. In the Indexes and abstracts we can find a brief summary, Author, Title, Place of publication of articles. Primary sources (Journals and Reports) and Secondary sources (Textbooks) also provide information about the problem of concern of the searching researcher.

To collect relevant source of information follow the below instructions

- Read headings carefully to know about the whole paper
- Read abstracts for the extract summary of the paper
- Read conclusion, to see the results of the study
- Read reference pages to find more sources related to that topic of interest.

The Process

Read the abstract and conclusion then the whole paper again and again. Try to take some notes soon after reading the articles and describe articles you have read by a summary. Description summary includes the following: Relationships between sources, Major themes and concepts of the study and any gaps and disagreements. Use mind maps or literature matrix while reading sources in order to understand theory, concepts and the relationships between them.

Literature matrix is an organizational tool which is very much used to display the relationship or common attributes of the studies e.g. table, chart or flow chart.

Mind map is an organizational tool which is very much used to visualize the relationship between themes.

Structure of the Literature Review

Identify the key themes and organize the concepts and documents in accordance with the key themes or use the literature matrix. Then the researcher can integrate the information by:

- Synthesis of key concepts
- Using helpful phrases to integrate key concepts
- Using direct quotations (cite the author, date and page number of the quote)
- Paraphrasing (acknowledge with a citation).

FURTHER READING

1. Fraenkel JR, Wallen NE. How to design and evaluate research in education (6th ed.). Boston, MA: McGraw Hill, 2006.
2. Hart C. Doing a literature search: A comprehensive guide for the social sciences. Thousand Oaks. CA: Sage; 2001.
3. Koh ET, Owen WL. Research Problem and Literature Review. In: Introduction to Nutrition and Health Research. Springer, Boston, MA, 2000.
4. Ridley D. The Literature Review: A step-by-step guide for students, (Los Angeles: Sage), 2008.

Research Design

RESEARCH DESIGN

Research design is not related to any particular method of collecting data or any particular type of data. Any research design can, in principle, use any type of data collection method and can use either quantitative or qualitative data. Research design refers to the structure of an enquiry: it is a logical matter rather than a logistical one. Research design is the framework that has been created to find answers to research questions.

Following are few definitions of Research design:

Ackoff: "It is the process of making decisions before the situation arises in which the decisions are to be carried out after for control".

According to Green and Tull, "It is the specification of techniques and processes for obtaining the information required. It is the over-all operational pattern or framework of the project which states what data is to be gathered from which source by what processes".

Miller: "Researcher Design is a planned sequence of the entire process involved in the conducting of as research study".

David J Luck and Ronald S Rubin: It is the determination and statement of the general research approach or approach followed for the specific task. It is the heart of planning. If the design sticks to the research objective, it will guarantee that the client's needs will be served.

EA Suchaman: "It is a series of guidelines or steps to keep one in right path".

A traditional research design is a blueprint or detailed plan for how a research study is to be completed—operationalizing variables so they can be measured, selecting a sample of interest to study, collecting data to be used as a basis for testing hypotheses, and analysing the results (Thyer 1993).

In the search for truth, basically researchers ask two fundamental types of research questions.

1. What and how is happening? Descriptive/Exploratory research/Quantitative.
2. Why it is happening? Explanatory/Confirmatory research/Qualitative.

Exploratory research—it is a type of research which seeks to generate a posteriori hypotheses by analyzing a collected data and mainly looking for potential relations between the variables. It is also possible to have an idea about a relation between variables but to lack knowledge of the direction and strength of the relation (potential cause-effect). If the researcher does not have any specific hypotheses before starting of the study, the study is exploratory with respect to the variables in question. The advantage of exploratory research is that it is easier to make new discoveries due to the less stringent methodological restrictions. Here, the researcher does not want to miss a potentially interesting relation and therefore aims to minimize the probability of rejecting a real effect or relation; this probability is sometimes referred to as β and the associated error is of type II. In other words, if the researcher simply wants to see whether some measured variables could be related, he would want to increase the chances of finding a significant result by lowering the threshold of what is deemed to be significant.

Confirmatory research—it is a type of research which tests priori hypotheses—outcome predictions are made before the measurement phase of the study begins. Such a priori hypotheses are usually derived from a theory or the results of previous studies mostly from exploratory research. The advantage of confirmatory research is that the result of this research is more meaningful, in the sense that it is much harder to claim that a certain result is generalizable beyond the data set. The reason for this is that in confirmatory research, the researcher ideally strives to reduce the probability of falsely reporting a coincidental result as meaningful. This probability is known as α-level or the probability of a type I error.

Exploratory and confirmatory research both complement each other because researches always start without any idea about the problem so that should be observed to make any hypothesis (Fig. 5.1).

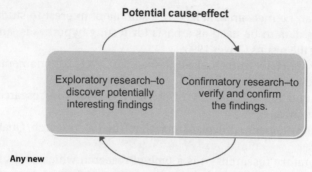

Figure 5.1: Exploratory and confirmatory research.

JW Tukey states in his renowned work, we need both exploratory and confirmatory approaches because "Finding the question is often more important than finding the answer".

Research design is different from the method by which data are collected. Failing to distinguish research design from research method leads to poor evaluation of research designs, e.g. A researcher may simply equating cross-sectional designs with questionnaires, or case studies with participant observation.

MEANING OF RESEARCH DESIGN

The central role of research design is to minimize the chance of drawing incorrect causal inferences from data. Design is a logical task undertaken to ensure that the evidence collected enables us to answer questions or to test theories as unambiguously as possible. When designing research it is essential that we identify the type of evidence required to answer the research question in a convincing way. While addressing a research question, it is essential that the question should be analyzed in the following possible ways which will make deciding of possible design as meaningful as possible.

- What is all the study about?
- Why is the study being done?
- Where will the study be carried out?
- What type of data is required?
- Where can the required data for the study be found?
- What periods of time will the study include? What will be the sample design?
- What techniques of data collection will be used?

- How will the data be analyzed?
- In what style will the report be prepared?

COMPONENTS OF RESEARCH DESIGN

Analyzing the research question from various angles help in identifying components of research design and take the researcher deeper into the research question to make the understanding clearer. Research design is basically a choice of the researcher about the components of the study and the selection of research components is done based on the consideration of the objectives and hypotheses of the study. Equally, Inappropriate choice of components may lead to a poor design with potential problems such as lack of precision, measurement errors and poor interpretation of the hypothesis testing.

Study design: There are many study designs in quantitative and qualitative research. Study designs in each paradigm are appropriate for finding different things. Quantitative study designs are specific, well structured, have been tested for their validity and reliability and intended to find out the extent of the variation and diversity (e.g. experimental study design, non-experimental study design, etc.). Study designs in qualitative research are less specific and precise, and do not have the same structural depth and intended to explore things in detail (e.g. case study, historical research, etc.). Figure 5.2 Various types of research designs are grouped based on the operational components of research. The reader should not confuse this classification with fundamental research enquiry designs like descriptive and exploratory.

Sampling design: It is a process of selection of a sample from population through various sampling methods for the study.

Observational design: It includes the methods of data collection. There are two types of data collection primary and secondary. Moreover it includes tools, procedure and measurement methods (e.g. Interview method, observation method, etc.).

Statistical design: It is the planning of appropriate statistical tests to be used to find the results from the collected data. Statistics is divided into major areas that are descriptive statistics and inferential statistics.

Operational design: It states the techniques by which procedures specified in the sampling, statistical and observational designs can be carried out by the researcher. It also includes execution of the tools, pilot testing and data entry and coding.

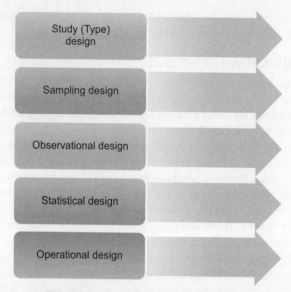

Figure 5.2: Components of research design.

NEED FOR RESEARCH DESIGN

Why do we need a research design? In the course of research process, for a smooth sailing of the various research operations step by step, and to maximize information with minimal expenditure of effort, time and money. In short, it is a method of advanced planning of a pathway in doing the work without deviating from the objective. Research design stands for advance planning of the methods to be adopted for collecting the relevant data and the techniques to be used in their analysis, keeping in view the objective of the research and the availability of staff, time and money. If the process of research satisfies the objective of the research in terms of knowledge addition, then it can be said that research design is good.

FEATURES FOR GOOD DESIGN

If the design for a specific question in the research satisfies certain criteria it is said to be a good design. The following are the good features of a research design:

- Flexible, appropriate, efficient and economical
- Minimizes bias in the study

- It should be free from confounding effect from extraneous variables
- Maximizes the reliability of the data
- Enhances the means of obtaining quantitative and qualitative information
- Fixes the availability and skills of the researcher and his staff
- A good statistical precision
- Favours the objective of the problem to be studied and the nature of the problem to be studied
- Facilitates the availability of time and money for the research work.

RESEARCH DESIGNS (TYPES)

Based on the methodology of conducting the research, various types of research designs that are used in health research. Figure 5.3 describes the all possible designs:

- Descriptive (e.g. case-study, naturalistic observation, survey)
- Correlational (e.g. case-control study, observational study)
- Semi-experimental (e.g. field experiment, quasi-experiment)
- Experimental (experiment with random assignment)

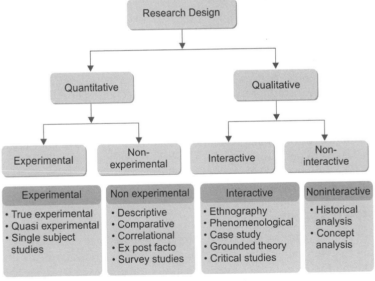

Figure 5.3: Types of research design.

- Review (literature review, systematic review)
- Meta-analytic (meta-analysis).

COMPARISON OF RESEARCH DESIGNS

Based on the components of research design the qualitative and quantitative research paradigms differ each other in principles. The differences are mentioned below in the table:

Table 5.1: Comparison of research designs

Part of the study	Qualitative	Quantitative
Study (Type) design	Flexible	Rigid
Sampling design	Non probability	Probability
Observational design	Unstructured instruments/tools	Structured instruments/tools
Statistical design	No pre-planned analysis	Planned analysis
Operational design	No fixed decisions	Methods are fixed/procedural

PRINCIPLES OF RESEARCH DESIGN

Apart from being a good design to the question in concern, specific to the exploratory research, a good design should satisfy following three principles though general principles for each type of design vary. Three principles of experimental designs are (According to Professor Fisher):

1. Principle of replication: The ability to repeat the experiment. Replication is introduced in order to increase the precision of a study.
2. Principle of randomization: Provides protection against the effects of extraneous factors.
3. Principle of local control: Shows the extraneous factor, the known source of variability, is made to vary deliberately over as wide a range as necessary and this needs to be done in such a way that the variability it causes can be measured and hence eliminated from the experimental error.

EFFECTIVE DESIGN

For a design to be an effective one for the intended question, research needs to be structured in such a way that the evidence also bears on alternative or contradictory explanations and enables the researcher to identify which of the competing explanation is most compelling empirically. The researchers must not simply look for evidence that supports the favorite theory what they hold. The researchers should also look for evidence that has the potential to disprove the preferred explanations.

CLINICAL STUDY DESIGN

To introduce the types of research designs in health research, this section narrates about the various questions in clinical research problems. **Clinical study design** is the formulation of trials and experiments, as well as observational studies in medical, clinical and other types of research involving human beings.

Types of designs for clinical studies:

Treatment studies	Observational studies

Treatment or Intervention Studies

Randomized controlled trial: Allocation of the subjects to the different treatment groups of a trial is done through proper randomization process to know the truth by a process of chance. Subjects in the trials are not limited to humans but may include animals, and other relevant things involved in testing.

Blind trial: The subjects and the experimenter who gives the intervention do not know about the details of the research. Blinding avoids observer and selection bias which prevents manipulation. Blinding and randomization where involved are the highest form of experimental design which eliminates bias and expected to test true cause-effect of variables of interest.

Non-blind trial: Subjects and the person who does measurement know about the purpose of the research. This may lead to more bias.

Nonrandomized trial (quasi-experiment): Allocation of the subjects to the different treatment groups of a trial is not done through proper randomization process.

Interrupted time series design (measures on a sample or a series of samples from the same population are obtained several times before and after a manipulated event or a naturally occurring event)—considered a type of quasi-experiment.

As a sub-group of interventional experimental designs, the following three designs are named based on the assumption of researcher over of interest in question. These may be experimental or quasi-experimental designs.

Superiority trials are designed to demonstrate that one treatment is more effective than a given reference treatment. This type of study design is often used to test the effectiveness of a treatment compared to placebo or to the currently best available treatment, e.g. McKenzie mobilization is better than conventional exercise program for chronic low back pain.

Non-inferiority trials are designed to demonstrate that a treatment is at least not appreciably less effective than a given reference treatment. This type of study design is often employed when comparing a new treatment to an established medical standard of care, in situations where the new treatment is cheaper, safer or more convenient than the reference treatment and would therefore be preferable if not appreciably less effective, e.g. laser therapy is equally effective as compared to intra-lesional injection for chronic wound healing.

Equivalence trials are designed to demonstrate that two treatments are equally effective. When using "parallel groups", each patient receives one treatment; in a "crossover study", each patient receives several treatments but in different order, e.g. Eficacy of interferential therapy and TENS in lumbar radiculopathy patients.

Observational Studies

Observational study designs are otherwise called as epidemiologic study designs and are predominantly used to study exposure-outcome relationship. Observational study designs involve prospective and retrospective cohorts, ecological, cross-sectional, case-control, case-crossover designs.

Cohort study: It identifies a group of patients who are already taking a particular treatment or have an exposure, follow them forward over time, and then compare their outcomes with a similar group that has not been affected by the treatment or exposure being studied.
- Prospective cohort-forward over time
- Retrospective cohort-backward over time

Time series study: Observations are done continuously for a period of time.

Case-control study: Patients who already have a specific condition are compared with people who do not have the condition. The term retrospective study is sometimes used as another term for a case-control study, is however often misleading, and should be avoided as other research designs are also retrospective in orientation.

Cross-sectional study: Describe the relationship between diseases and other factors at one point in time in a defined population.

Community survey: It is a type of cross-sectional study only, targeting a population belong to a particular community and can be studied for many variables in interest.

Ecological study: An ecological study is an observational study in which at least one variable is measured at the group level. This type of study is especially appropriate for initial investigation of causal hypothesis. Examples of group-level measures include the incidence rate of cancer among a specific population, the mean level of blood pressure of patients seen at a clinic and the average sunlight exposure at specific geographic location.

A longitudinal study assesses research subjects over two or more points in time, but a cross-sectional study assesses research subjects at only one point in time (so case-control, cohort, and randomized studies are not cross-sectional).

FURTHER READING

1. Carr LT. The strengths and weaknesses of quantitative and qualitative research: What method for nursing? Journal of Advanced Nursing, 1994;20(4), 716-721.
2. Creswell JW. Research design: Qualitative and quantitative approaches. Thousand Oaks, CA: SAGE Publications, 1994.
3. Hartung DM, Touchette D. "Overview of clinical research design". American Journal of Health-System Pharmacy, 2009;66(4):398-408.
4. Hinotsu S. Selection of appropriate design in the development of interventional and observational research. Gan To Kagaku Ryoho, 2014; 41(4):405-09.
5. Leedy P, Ormrod J. Practical research: Planning and design (7th ed.). Upper Saddle River, NJ: Merrill Prentice Hall. Thousand Oaks: SAGE Publications, 2001.
6. Noordzij M, et al. "Study designs in clinical research." Nephron ClinPract, 2009;113(3):c218-21.

CHAPTER

6

Sampling Design and Sampling Distributions

SAMPLE DESIGN

Sample design or sampling is selecting a subset of units from a target population for the purpose of collecting information (Sampling method). The study of the total population is not possible in practical sense due to cost, time and other factors which are usually operative in the situation and stand in the way of studying the total population. So the concept of sampling has been introduced to make the research process economical and accurate. Moreover sampling is the fundamental to all statistical methodology. It is similar to assuming that a small piece of cake's taste will give individual the information about the taste of the cakes produced in that set. Thus purpose of sampling is to study a section of population assuming that it is representative for the issue of interest in the whole population.

DIFFERENT TYPES OF SAMPLE DESIGN

1. Probability sampling
2. Non-probability sampling
1. **Probability sampling:** It is a type of selection process in which every unit has equal chance of being selected so as to know that any information about a process can be learnt by chance if it is representative of the population. The main features of different types of random sampling are:
   - Simple random sampling: Subjects have equal chance of being selected.
   - Systematic random sampling: Started at random and picking every 'n'th element in succession.
   - Stratified random sampling: Population is divided into stratum/subpopulation and random sampling done on each stratum or group
   - Cluster random sampling: Whole population is divided into clusters and clusters are selected randomly (Fig. 6.1).
2. **Non-probability sampling:** Subjects are being selected at the convenience of the researcher or based on the purpose of the study. It is similar to subjects being selectively chosen to suit the results that we are expecting. But in reality in the actual population the result may be different. Hence, non-probability sampling does not unmask the reality about a topic of interest. The main features of different non-probability sampling are given in Figure 6.2:
   Convenience sampling: Subjects are selected to our convenience. For example: A person going in the street is chosen as he is conveniently near us to study.
   Purposive sampling: Usually one or more specific predefined groups are selected with some purpose in mind.
   Quota sampling: Selection is based on predefined sections in population, e.g. Proportional gender selection.
   Judgment sampling: Selection is based on the judgment of an expert which may dependant on investigators knowledge and professional judgment.

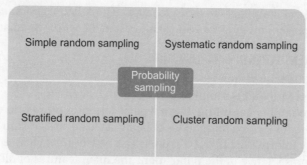

Figure 6.1: Probability sampling.

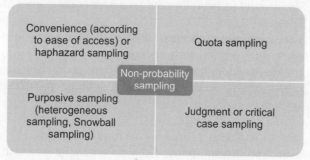

Figure 6.2: Non-probability sampling.

Difference between probability sampling and non-probability sampling is given in Table 6.1.

Table 6.1: Difference between Probability sampling and Non probability sampling

Probability sampling	Non-probability sampling
Unrestricted sampling (simple random sampling)	Unrestricted sampling (haphazard or convenience sampling)
Or	Or
Restricted sampling (stratified, cluster or systematic complex random sampling)	Restricted sampling (purposive sampling such as quota sampling, judgment sampling)
No representation bias	Bias is present
By chance	By convenience

CRITERIA FOR SELECTING SAMPLING PROCEDURE

Every step in research should be carefully executed and sampling as first step is no exception to this. There are every possible deviation in the result that may be effected if appropriate sampling procedure is not considered. Hence, while selecting a sampling procedure, researcher

must ensure that the procedure causes a relatively small sampling error and helps to control the systematic bias in a better way. It is important that the below mentioned criteria are verified for sampling procedures to be as effective as possible.

- Inappropriate sampling frame
- Defective measuring device
- Non-respondents
- Indeterminacy principle
- Natural bias in the reporting of data.

STEPS IN SAMPLING DESIGN

The following are the steps that shall be followed to make a decision on which type of sampling would suit the research topic undertaken by a researcher.

- Type of universe
- Sampling unit
- Sampling frame (source list)
- Sample size
- Parameters of interest
- Financial constraints
- Procedure of sampling.

CHARACTERISTICS OF GOOD SAMPLE DESIGN

The intended notion in a research can be achieved only if sample characteristics are good enough to satisfy the purpose of the research question.

- A truly representative sample from the population
- Small sampling error
- No systematic bias: Bias in sampling is a systematic error in sampling procedures that lead to a distortion in the result of the study
- Fewer funds used
- A good generalizability of the results.

SAMPLING ERROR

A sampling error is a statistical error that occurs when researcher does not select a sample that represents the entire population of data. In analyzing the data, the results section need look into the facets of deviations to identify if the deviation could be due to the sampling error. Hence every possible error like frame, chance, and response need to be eliminated by determining appropriate sample size (Fig. 6.3).

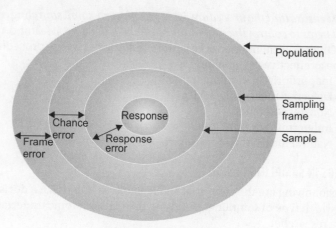

Figure 6.3: Sampling error.

Sampling error = Frame error + Chance error + Response error
Total error = Sampling error + Non-sampling or measurement error

IMPLICATIONS FOR SAMPLE DESIGN

The major implications of a proper sample design are mentioned below:

- Sample size selection
- Selection of sample from population
- Less error
- Saves time, energy and money

SAMPLING FUNDAMENTAL DEFINITIONS

Details about the sample and related terminologies are important to effect proper method of sampling. Table 6.2 mentions about the common terminologies used in research about sampling. Knowledge about the terminologies also help researcher in rightful reporting about the study.

Table 6.2: Sampling fundamental definitions

Universe/Population (finite or infinite)	All the individuals or objects which are to be studied.
Sampling units	A sampling unit is one of the units into which an aggregate is divided for the purpose of sampling, each unit being regarded as individual and indivisible when the selection is made.

Contd...

Contd...

Sampling frame	It is the source material or device from which a **sample** is drawn. It is a list of all those within a population who can be **sampled**.
Sampling design	Selecting a subset of units from a target population for the purpose of collecting information (**Sampling method**).
Statistic/Parameter	Measures such as mean, median, mode or the like ones from samples are called statistic(s) as they describe the characteristics of a sample. But when such measures describe the characteristics of a population, they are known as parameter(s). Parameter (Population characteristic) e.g. μ, σ, P, median, percentiles, etc. Statistic (sample characteristic), e.g. x, s, sample proportion, etc.
Sampling error	A sampling error is a statistical error that occurs when researcher does not select a sample that represents the entire population of data.
Precision	In statistics, precision is the reciprocal of the variance. It refers to how close estimates from different samples are to each other. For example, the standard error is a measure of precision.
Confidence interval	It is a type of interval estimate (of a population parameter) that is computed from the observed data. A Confidence Interval is a range of values we are fairly sure our true value lies in.
Point estimator	A point estimator is a formula that uses sample data to calculate a single number (a sample statistic) that can be used as an estimate of a population parameter. e.g. $\bar{x}$, s *to calculate* μ, σ.

DISTRIBUTIONS

The **distribution** of a **statistical** data set or a population is a description of all the possible values of the data, e.g. **distribution** of categorical data is number or percentage of individuals in each group. Hence sampling directly affects through the inferences taken from the results of the study which are represented by distributions in the study.

SAMPLING DISTRIBUTIONS

The concept of a sampling distribution is perhaps the most basic concept in inferential statistics. The different types are:
- The sampling distribution of the mean
- The sampling distribution of the difference between means

- The sampling distribution of r
- The sampling distribution of a proportion.

Population, Sample and Sampling Distributions

Population distributions	4,6,8,10		
Sample distributions	Sample A: 4,6,10	Sample B: 4,6,8	Sample C: 6,8,10
Sampling distributions of Mean	6.66	6.00	8.00

The above tabular column represents the distributions of a variable of interest in a study and analysis of the sample distributions. A small representation of a variable of interest informs about the distributions and related analytics about the variable. The reader can refer to related contents for further information.

CENTRAL LIMIT THEOREM

The central limit theorem states that: *Given a population with a finite mean μ and a finite non-zero variance σ2, the sampling distribution of the mean approaches a normal distribution with a mean of μ and a variance of σ2/N as N, the sample size, increases.* **Example of the Central Limit Theorem in Practice: When** Roll 30 dice and calculate the average (sample mean) of the numbers that you get on each die. Now repeat this experiment 1000 times each time rolling 30 dice and computing a new sample mean. Plot a histogram of the 1000 sample means that you have obtained. This plot will look approximately normal.

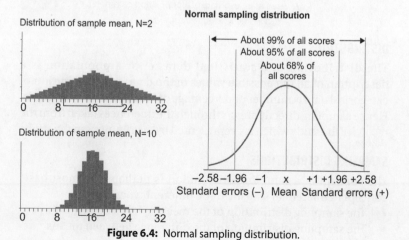

Figure 6.4: Normal sampling distribution.

Given below are the examples of various types of sampling distributions all of which satisfies central limit theorem as the sample size increases.

SAMPLING DISTRIBUTION OF MEAN/Z DISTRIBUTION

Sampling distribution of mean refers to the probability distribution of all the possible means of random samples of a given size that we take from a population. If samples are taken from a normal population, the 'z' is calculated by the formula below:

$$z = \frac{\bar{x} - \mu}{\sigma_p / \sqrt{n}}$$

SAMPLING DISTRIBUTION OF PROPORTION/BINOMIAL DISTRIBUTION

Usually the statistics of attributes correspond to the conditions of a binomial distribution that tends to become normal distribution as n becomes larger and larger. If p represents the proportion of defectives, i.e. of successes and q the proportion of non-defectives, i.e. of failures (or q = 1 - p) and if p is treated as a random variable, then the sampling distribution of proportion of successes has a mean = p with standard deviation = p × q n, where n is the sample size.

$$z = \frac{\hat{p} - p}{\sqrt{(p \cdot q)/n}}$$

SAMPLING DISTRIBUTION OF MEAN/'t' DISTRIBUTION

The variable t differs from z in the sense that we use sample standard deviation in the calculation of t, whereas we use standard deviation of population in the calculation of z. There is a different t distribution for every possible sample size, i.e. for different degrees of freedom. The degrees of freedom for a sample of size n is $n - 1$. As the sample size gets larger, the shape of the t distribution becomes approximately equal to the normal distribution.

$$t = \left(\bar{X} - \mu \right) / \left(\sigma_s / \sqrt{n} \right)$$

THE SAMPLING DISTRIBUTION OF THE DIFFERENCE BETWEEN MEANS/*F DISTRIBUTIONS*

Two independent normal populations, having the same variance. The calculated value of *F* from the sample data is compared with the corresponding table value of *F* and if the former is equal to or exceeds the latter, then we infer that the null hypothesis of the variances being equal cannot be accepted. We shall make use of the *F* ratio in the context of hypothesis testing and also in the context of ANOVA technique.

$(\sigma_{p1})^2 = (\sigma_{p2})^2$, the ratio $F = (\sigma_{s1})^2/(\sigma_{s2})^2$, where $(\sigma_{s1})^2 = \Sigma (\overline{X}_{1i} - \overline{X}_1)^2/n_1 - 1$ and $(\sigma_{s2})^2 = \Sigma (\overline{X}_{2i} - \overline{X}_2)^2/n_2 - 1$ has an F distribution with $n_1 - 1$ and $n_2 - 1$ degrees of freedom.

SAMPLING DISTRIBUTION - *CHI-SQUARE DISTRIBUTION*

Distribution is not symmetrical and all the values are positive with $(n - 1)$ degrees of freedom.

Chi-square distribution is encountered when we deal with collections of values that involve adding up squares.

$$\chi^2 = \sum_{i=1}^{k} \frac{(O_i - E_i)^2}{E_i}$$

SAMPLE SIZE CALCULATION

Sample size and calculation of sample size is an important issue in research. When a researcher selects a sample it should be representative of the population and very much precise enough to avoid uncertainty. As far as unrepresentative sample is concerned it may lead to biased conclusions and when precision is concerned if the sample is large, the smaller the margin of uncertainty (narrow confidence interval).

To calculate a sample size, the researcher may need some rough idea about the degree of precision or uncertainty. And many sample size calculations also require an effect size value to calculate required sample size. Thus, sample size calculation in a particular study depends mainly on:

- The anticipated clinical difference between the alternative treatments/effect size
- The level of statistical significance ($p<.05$); One and two-sided significance tests

- Type I error (α) (Conventionally $\alpha = 0.05$ is often used)
- The chance of detecting the anticipated clinical difference
- Power ($1 - \beta$) (Conventionally a minimum power of 80% is required).

In estimating the number of patients required (sample size) for a study, one should identify a single major outcome which is regarded as the primary outcome measure for comparing treatment mean differences. In physiotherapy clinical trials this will be a measure such as pain severity, disability, balance score, or a quality of life score. However, often there is more than one outcome measure of interest within a study. If one of this outcome measures is regarded as more important than the other one, it is named as the primary outcome or endpoint and sample-size is calculated based on that. But most of the times a problem arises when there are several outcome measures and all are considered equally important in the study. In that situation the commonly adopted approach is to calculate the sample-size estimates for each outcome measure in turn, and then select the largest number as the sample size required for the study. Among all the factors responsible the following sections discusses about two of the most important ones, one the statistical significance and another situation where there is no effect size for a particular treatment from previous studies.

Sample Size and Interpretation of Statistical Significance

Suppose, from a previous study, if the results of an observed treatment difference is 'not statistically significant', it does not imply that there is 'no clinically important difference between the treatments'. For example, if the sample size was too small in the study trial the researcher may obtain a not significant p-value even when a clinically relevant difference is truly present. Hence it is of more of importance to consider sample size and power when interpreting statements about 'non-significant' results. In particular, if the power of the test was very low the researcher can conclude from a non-significant result that the question of treatment differences remains unresolved in the study. And as a next attempt the researcher may propose in his study to increase the sample size and so as to study the true effect further. This may reduce the degree of uncertainty or increase the precision. Deciding on the sample size involve power calculation represented as ($1 - \beta$).

Pilot Study and Sample Size

Sometimes researchers conduct and use the pilot study results to calculate the sample size which is contradicted by many authors. Two important considerations should be kept in mind when using pilot study for estimation of sample size:

1. The final sample size should only ever be adjusted upwards, never downwards

2. One should only use pilot results in order to improve the design features which are independent of the treatment variable. For example: If treatments are to be compared using a t-test, then for sample-size calculation standard deviation will be used whose value may be amended following the pilot phase and then potentially used to revise the sample size upwards.

FORMULAE FOR SAMPLE SIZE CALCULATIONS

Formulae for sample size calculations vary based on the knowledge about the target population.

If the target population is unknown	If the target population is known
$$n = \dfrac{Z_{\frac{\alpha}{2}}^2 \, p(1-p)}{e^2}$$ where: $P = 0.05$ $Z_{0.025} = 1.96$ $e = \text{error } (.01)$ $n = 1825$	$$n = \dfrac{NZ_{\frac{\alpha}{2}}^2 \, p(1-p)}{e^2(N-1) + Z_{\frac{\alpha}{2}}^2 \, p(1-p)}$$

SAMPLE SIZE FOR DIFFERENT TYPE OF STUDIES

1. **Sample size for simple prevalence (proportions and percentages) studies (Table 6.3).**

   The sample size needed for a prevalence study depends on how precisely (the amount of error in a measurement) **a researcher wants to measure the prevalence** (proportion of people who have the condition).

   Decide on the acceptable margin of error: For an exploratory study, for example, a margin of error of ±10% might be perfectly acceptable. Less the margin of error more the sample we need. From Table 6.3 it can be seen that with less margin of error in a given population, the sample size increases. Whereas higher the margin of error the sample size decreases.

Is study population finite or infinite: In a finite population, the sample size is smaller

Table 6.3: Sample sizes for prevalence studies

Acceptable margin of error	Size of population					
	Large	5000	2500	1000	500	200
±20%	24	24	24	23	23	22
±15%	43	42	42	41	39	35
±10%	96	94	93	88	81	65
±7.5%	171	165	160	146	127	92
±5%	384	357	333	278	217	132
±3%	1067	880	748	516	341	169

2. Sample sizes for studies comparing proportions between two groups (Table 6.4)

   Decide on the difference of prevalence between the groups
   Sample sizes are bigger (per group) when the condition has a prevalence of 50% in one of the groups. As the prevalence in one group goes towards 0% or 100%, the sample size requirement falls.

   Decide the power of the study (80%, 90% or 95%), e.g. A study with 90% power is 90% likely to discover the difference between the groups if such a difference exists.

Table 6.4: Sample sizes for studies comparing proportions between two groups

Difference between the groups	Prevalence in one group 50%		Prevalence in one group 25%		Prevalence in one group 10%	
	Power		Power		Power	
	90%	95%	90%	95%	90%	95%
5%	2134	2630	1714	2110	957	2134
10%	538	661	460	563	286	538
15%	240	293	216	264	146	240
20%	134	163	128	155	92	134
25%	85	103	85	103	65	85
30%	58	70	61	73	49	58

Sample Sizes for Comparing the Means of Two Groups (Independent)

Decide the smallest clinically significant difference, e.g. 2.5 on a 11 point numerical pain rating scale.

Convert the smallest clinically significant difference to standard deviation (SD) units.

If Expected mean value for the control or group is – E.g. 6

Highest typical value- 8; lowest typical value-2, then

Approximate SD = (Highest typical value — lowest typical value) ÷ 4 (Since most values will be within ±2 SD of the average)

$$(8-2 \div 4) = 1.5$$

Convert the minimum difference to be detected to standard deviation units - dividing it by the standard deviation. For example: In studying the response of heat treatment to a tendinitis amongst a sample of Indians and Pakistanis living in America measured on a pain rating scale, if the researcher keeps the difference that need to be detected as very small, then the sample size increases.

Minimum difference detected ÷ standard deviation

$$2.5 \div 1.5 = 1.66$$

[Sample size required for comparing the mean values of two groups If researcher intended using a nonparametric test, multiply the sample size by 1.16]

Sample sizes for comparing the means of two groups (independent) are given in Table 6.5.

Table 6.5: Sample sizes for comparing the means of two groups (independent)

Difference to be detected (SD units)	N in each group 90% power	N in each group 95% power
2	6	7
1.5	10	12
1.4	11	14
1.3	13	16
1.25	14	17
1.2	15	19
1.1	18	22
1	22	26
0.9	26	33
0.8	33	41
0.75	38	47
0.7	43	54

Contd...

Contd...

Difference to be detected (SD units)	N in each group 90% power	N in each group 95% power
0.6	59	73
0.5	85	104
0.4	132	163
0.3	234	289
0.25	337	416
0.2	526	650

Sample Sizes for Comparing the Means of Two Groups (Paired/Dependent) (Table 6.6)

Decide the smallest clinically significant difference, e.g. 2.5 on a 11 point numerical pain rating scale

Imagine, in the same example above, if a treatment modality is tested as pre and post-test design in either Indians or Pakistanis, then sample size calculation for such a group would be:

Convert the smallest clinically significant difference to standard deviation units.

biggest typical positive difference - 5 point reduction of pain

biggest typical negative difference - 2 points increase in pain

Approximate SD = (biggest typical positive difference — biggest typical negative difference) ÷ 4

$$(5-2) \div 4 = 0.75$$

Table 6.6: Sample sizes for comparing the means of two groups (paired/dependent)

Difference to be detected (SD units)	N required for 90% power	N required for 95% power
2	3	4
1.5	5	6
1.4	6	7
1.3	7	8
1.25	7	9
1.2	8	10
1.1	9	11
1	11	13
0.9	13	17
0.8	17	21
0.75	19	24
0.7	22	27

Contd...

Contd...

Difference to be detected (SD units)	N required for 90% power	N required for 95% power
0.6	30	37
0.5	43	52
0.4	66	82
0.3	117	145
0.25	169	208
0.2	263	325

Sample Size for Correlations between Two Variables (Numeric Scale)

Squaring of a correlation gives the proportion of variation in one variable that is linked to variation in another variable. For example, there is a correlation of 0.7, the variation is 0.49, that is 50% approximately.

Table 6.7: Sample size for correlations between two variables (numeric scale)

% Shared variation	Correlation	Sample size 90% power	Sample size 95% power
10%	0.32	99	121
20%	0.45	48	59
30%	0.55	30	37
40%	0.63	22	27
50%	0.71	16	20

Sample size for scale reliability studies (Cronbach's alpha coefficient)

Decide on the reliability at which the scale would be unacceptable (less than 0.6 for development; less than 0.8 for decision making about people).

Decide on the minimum reliability (0.86 for development; 0.9 for decision making about people).

Decide the number of items in the scale.

Table 6.8: Sample size for scale reliability studies

Number of items	Minimum acceptable reliability	Minimum desired reliability	Number for 90% power	Number for 95% power
5	0.6	0.7	136	171
		0.8	27	34
10	0.6	0.7	109	138
		0.8	22	28

Contd...

Contd...

Number of items	Minimum acceptable reliability	Minimum desired reliability	Number for 90% power	Number for 95% power
15	0.6	0.7	102	128
		0.8	21	26
20	0.6	0.7	98	124
		0.8	21	26
5	0.8	0.9	36	45
		0.95	10	13
10	0.8	0.9	31	39
		0.95	9	11
15	0.8	0.9	30	37
		0.95	9	11
20	0.8	0.9	29	36
		0.95	9	11

SOFTWARE FOR SAMPLE SIZE CALCULATIONS

1. Biostat (2001). Power and Precision: Release 2.1. Englewood, NJ.
2. Lenth RV (2006). Java Applets for Power and Sample Size. URL: http://www.stat.uiowa.edu/ ~rlenth/Power.
3. National Council for Social Studies (2005). Power Analysis and Sample Size Software (PASS): Version 2005. NCSS Statistical Software, Kaysville, UT.
4. SAS Institute (2004). Getting Started with the SAS Power and Sample Size Application: Version 9.1. SAS Institute, Cary, NC.
5. StataCorp (2007). Stata Statistical Software: Release 10. College Station, TX.
6. Statistical Solutions (2006).nQuery Adviser: Version 6.0. Saugus, MA.

Books and References for Sample Size Calculation

Resources for sample size calculations are given for further understanding:

1. Chow SC, Shao J, Wang H. Sample Size Calculations in Clinical Research, 2nd editionn. Marcel Dekker, New York, 2008.

2. Machin D, Campbell MJ. Design of Studies for Medical Research, John Wiley and Sons, Chichester, 2005 .

3. A'Hern RP. Sample size tables for exact single stage phase II designs. Statistics in Medicine, 2001;20:859–866.

4. Van Belle G. Statistical Rules of Thumb. John Wiley and Sons, Chichester, 2002.

5. Cohen J. Statistical Power Analysis for the Behavioral Sciences, 2nd edition. Lawrence Earlbaum, New Jersey, 1988.

ONLINE SAMPLE SIZE CALCULATORS/RESOURCES

1. http://home.clara.net/sisa/sampshlp.htm
2. http://statpages.org/index.html#Power
3. http://hedwig.mgh.harvard.edu/sample_size/size.html
4. http://statpages.org/javasta2.html
5. The **Graph Pad** website (http://graphpad.com/welcome.htm)
6. Sample-sizecalculator**StatMate**-http://graphpad.com/StatMate/statmate.htm.
7. Windows sample size calculator -http://homepage.usask.ca/~jic956/work/MorePower.html
8. Epicalc 2000 includes sample size calculation- http://www.brixtonhealth.com/epicalc.html
9. Free calculator for the **Palm** - http://www.bobwheeler.com/stat/SSize/ssize.html

FURTHER READING

1. Charan J, Biswas T. How to Calculate Sample Size for Different Study Designs in Medical Research? *Indian Journal of Psychological Medicine*, 2013;35(2), 121–126. http://doi.org/10.4103/0253-7176.116232.

2. Das S, et al. "Sample size calculation: Basic principles." Indian J Anaesth 2016;60(9):652-656.

3. Lavrakas P. Encyclopedia of Survey Research Methods, 2008.

4. Lohr S. Sampling: Design and Analysis. California. Duxbury Press, 1999; p512.

5. Noordzij M, et al. "Sample size calculations." Nephron ClinPract 2011; 118(4): c319-323.

6. Zodpey SP. Sample size and power analysis in medical research. Indian J Dermatol Venereol Leprol 2004;70(2):123-128.

CHAPTER 7

Measurement, Scaling, Data Collection and Processing

MEASUREMENT AND SCALING

In any research, measurements of the intended changes and findings are very important to analyze the directions or trend of the involved variables. This will help to make conclusions about the question asked in research. Measurement can be defined as a standardized process of assigning numbers or other symbols to observations or responses according to some set of rules. Symbols may be mathematical symbols or word codes depending on the type of research that is undertaken whether qualitative or quantitative. Most of the measurements are done in scales and, Scaling is considered as the extension of measurement. Basically there are four levels of scales classified based on the characteristics of variables in question—Nominal, Ordinal, Interval, and Ratio Scales.

CHARACTERISTICS OF SCALING

The four levels of scales- Nominal, Ordinal, Interval, and Ratio Scales

• Description: ("yes" or "no"/"agree" or "disagree")
• Order: (1 is less than 5)

- Distance: (absolute differences expressed in units)
- Origin: (if there is a unique beginning or true zero point for the scale)

"Each scaling property builds on the previous one."

Scaling Properties				
Scale	Description	Order	Distance	Origin
Nominal	Yes	No	No	No
Ordinal	Yes	Yes	No	No
Interval	Yes	Yes	Yes	No
Ratio	Yes	Yes	Yes	Yes

LEVELS OF SCALES (TABLE 7.1)

Nominal scale: Datasets generated for a sample containing nominal data can be two or more categories (Ref examples above). Hence, this is termed as categorical data which is not ordered.

Which of the following exercise program satisfies you a lot? The patients may anyone of the following:

- Stretching exercise program
- Balance training program
- Home exercise program
- Strengthening exercise program ✓

Ordinal scale: The data set generated in a sample containing ordinal data will be ordered in an ascending or descending manner. Hence it is called ranked categorical data.

Please rank the following list according to your degree of liking for each.

Table 7.1: Levels of scales

Level	Example	Statistics
Nominal scale	Yes/no, Female/male Either/or, racial groups	Counting (frequencies, mode)
Ordinal scale	Rankings, level of income Any hierrarchial	Counting and ordering (frequencies, mode, median, Range)
Interval scale	Likert scale, number of siblings, no of motor bikes	Descriptive statistics (mean, median, mode, standard deviation)
Ratio scale	Blood pressure value, height, weight	Descriptive statistics (mean, median, mode, standard deviation)

(Assign most preferred exercise program rank = 1 and your least preferred exercise program rank = 4)

- Stretching exercise program-2
- Balance training program-3
- Home exercise program-4
- Strengthening exercise program-1

Interval Scale

Please indicate your degree of liking of each of the exercise program on the following list by checking the appropriate position on the scale with a tick mark. The final data set represents the number of events when calculated on the whole for a given sample, and the dataset exhibits itself in a numerical value. Hence it is also termed as discrete numerical data.

	Dislike a lot	Dislike	Neutral	Like	Like a lot
Stretching exercise program			✓		
Balance training program				✓	
Home exercise program	✓				
Strengthening exercise program				✓	

Ratio scale: The data set containing a sample with ratio scale are usually in numbers and hence also called as continuous numerical data.

Please divide and distribute 100 points given among each of the following exercise program according to your degree of liking for each:

- Stretching exercise program (20 points)
- Balance training program (30 points)
- Home exercise program (10 points)
- Strengthening exercise program (40 points)

CLASSIFICATION OF SCALING

The classification of scaling is based on: The way a variable is classified as a belonging to a particular scale depends on the below mentioned factors

- Subject orientation, Response form (open/closed), Degree of subjectivity, Scale properties (nominal, ordinal, interval or ratio), Number of dimensions (unidimenstional/multidimenstional)
- Scale construction techniques
  1. Arbitrary approach—rely on researcher's insight and competence
  2. Consensus approach—Thurstone differential scale
  3. Item analysis approach—Likert's summated scale
  4. Cumulative scales—Guttman's scalogram
  5. Factor scales—Osgoods semantic differential, multidimensional scale

THE SCALING TECHNIQUES (TABLE 7.2)

- **The comparative scales (*non-metric scaling*)**
- **The non-comparative scales (*monadic or metric* scales)**

Table 7.2: The scaling techniques

Types of comparative scales	Types of non- comparative scales
Paired comparison Rank order Constant sum Q-sort and other procedures	Continuous rating scales Itemized rating scales • Likert scale • Semantic differential scale • Stapel scale • Thurstone scale

Paired Comparison

It is a comparative scaling technique wherein the respondent is shown two objects at the same time and is asked to select one according to the defined criterion. The resulting data are ordinal in nature. It uses the assumption of transitivity. It is effective when the number of objects are limited because it requires the direct comparison.

Example

Brand 1	Brand 2	Preference
Tapsi stimulator	Electromed stimulator	
Striker stimulator	Tapsi stimulator	
Biomed stimulator	Electromed stimulator	
Striker stimulator	Biomed stimulator	

Rank Order Scale

In this rank order scale the numbers are assigned to the objects to determine the relative extent to which certain characteristic is possessed. It helps in identifying that whether the object has more or less of a characteristic as compared to another object, but does not tell about how much or less the characteristic is from the another.

Please rank the following search tools to find research literature in order (1—most preferred; 5—least preferred)

3	Google scholar
2	Pubmed
4	Biomed central
1	Cohrane
5	CINHAL

Constant Sum

It is a technique wherein the respondents are asked to allocate a constant sum of units, such as points, among the stimulus objects according to some specified criterion. Please divide and distribute 100 points given among each of the following exercise program according to your degree of liking for each:

Google scholar	20
Pubmed	20
Biomed central	15
Cohrane	35
CINHAL	10
Total	100

Continuous Rating Scales (Graphic Rating Scale)

It is a non-comparative scale technique wherein the respondents are asked to rate the stimulus objects by placing a mark appropriately on a line running from one extreme of the criterion to the other variable criterion, e.g. pain rating scales.

No pain--**worst pain**

0 10 20 30 40 50 60 70 80 90 100

Semantic Differential Scale

The Semantic Differential Scale is a seven-point rating scale used to derive the respondent's attitude towards the given object or event by asking him to select an appropriate position on a scale between two bipolar adjectives. The scale has properties of an interval scale.

How do you describe the hospitality in physiotherapy OPD?

1 2 3 4 5 6 7	
Empathic _____	Empathetic
Clean _____	Dirty
High quality _____	Low quality
Cold _____	Warm
Comfortable _____	Embarrassing
Innovative _____	Conservative

Likert's Scale

A Likert scale is a scale used to measure the attitude wherein the respondents are asked to indicate the level of agreement or disagreement with the statements related to the stimulus objects. The response for each individual statement is expressed on a category scale.

Each statement shall be evaluated on a scale of 1 to 5, e.g. Depression scale.

Since last four weeks I feel helpless most of the times:

1. Strongly disagree
2. Disagree
3. Neither agree nor disagree
4. Somewhat agree
5. Strongly agree

Stapel Scale

Stapel scale is a unipolar (one adjective) rating scale designed to measure the respondent's attitude towards the object or event. The scale is comprised of 10 categories ranging from –5 to +5 without any neutral point. A simplified version of the semantic differential scale in which a single adjective or descriptive phrase is used instead of bipolar adjectives. Characteristics 1. The scale measures both the direction and intensity of the attribute simultaneously

+5
+4
+3
+2
+1

Patient satisfaction

                –1
                –2
                –3
                –4
                –5

Sorting

The Q-Sort scaling is a Rank order scaling technique. It requires that respondents indicate their attitudes or beliefs by arranging items on the basis of perceived similarity or some other attribute. It is a useful technique for sorting relatively large numbers of objects quite quickly. A type of comparative scale where respondents are asked to sort between 60–90 objects usually.

Example: *Put these cards in the pockets next to the hospitals you would prefer to avail physiotherapy. You can put as many cards as you want or you can put no cards next to any hospital.*

Cards
LMSH hospital_____
Delta hospital _____
*United hospital*_____
*Mathew hospital*_____
*Swan hospital*_____

ADVANTAGES AND DISADVANTAGES OF RATING SCALES

Advantages and disadvantages of rating scales are provided in Table 7.3.

Table 7.3: Advantages and disadvantages of rating scales

Scale	Advantages	Disadvantages
Category scale	Flexible, easy	Ambiguous
Likert's scale	Easy	Individual score is difficult to interpret
Semantic differential scale	Easy to construct	Ordinal data
Staple scale	Easy to administer	Numerical data
Graphic scale	Easy for illiterates	No standard answer/ explanation
Constant sum scale	Interval scale	Difficult for illiterates

STRENGTHS OF SCALES

For a scale to be useful for research processes, it should be valid and reliable. Validity and reliability of a variable should be tested in all the domains.

- Validity
  - Content validity
  - Construct validity
  - Predictive validity
  - Concurrent validity
  - Face validity
- Reliability
  - Test-retest reliability, internal consistency
  - Split-half reliability
- Sensitivity and specificity

ERRORS IN MEASUREMENT

Errors in measurement can occur for various reasons. It is very important that errors are minimized as much possible so that the intention for which the research is carried out is achieved. Below mentioned are the some of the common errors in a research.

- Respondent error, e.g. bored/annoyed subject
- Situational error, e.g. presence of somebody
- Measurer error, e.g. calculation/coding error
- Instrumentation error, e.g. poor tool preparation
- Errors of observation
- Errors of non-observation (poor sampling frame, sampling error, non-response).

METHODS OF DATA COLLECTION

Various methods of collecting data are employed by the researcher and it begins after a research problem and research design has been finalised. There are two types of data collection primary and secondary. The data which are collected at source for the first time happen to be original in character, not subjected to any processing or manipulation is known as Primary data. It is basically collected by means of survey, observation or experimentation Table 7.4): If the data is already collected and used for analysis is called secondary data which is normally obtained from books, unpublished data or magazines.

Table 7.4: Methods of data collection

Primary data (data we collect)	Secondary data (data someone else has collected)
• Surveys • Focus groups • Questionnaires • Personal interviews • Experiments and observational study	• Country health departments • Vital Statistics – birth, death certificates • Hospital, clinic, school nurse records • Private and foundation databases • Surveillance data from state /central government programs, e.g. Census.
Limitations	**Limitations**
Researcher error Uniqueness Time and money Measurement error	Time of collection How? Reliable source Confounding bias Incomplete data set Consistency

DATA COLLECTION TOOLS

There are various tools or sources used to collect primary and secondary data. The tools have a specific purpose of translating the tools into specific questions/items related to the objectives of research and the information gathered in the appropriate form will form the data. The variables and their interrelationships are analyzed for testing the hypothesis of the research. A brief introduction of the important tools is given below (Table 7.5).

Table 7.5: Data collection tools

Tools of primary data	Tools of secondary data
Participatory methods	Files/records
Records and secondary data	Computer data bases
Observation	Industry or government reports
Surveys and interviews	Other reports or prior evaluations
Focus groups	Census data and household survey data
Use of mechanical devices	Electronic mailing lists
Case study method	Discussion groups
Diaries, journals, self-reported checklists	Documents (budgets, organizational
Expert judgment	charts, policies and procedures, maps,
Delphi technique	monitoring reports)
	Newspapers and television reports

Each of the above tools is used for a specific method of data gathering in research.

Observation Schedule

This is a form or sheet on which observations of an object or a phenomenon by the observers are recorded. The observation could be either structured or unstructured. The items to be observed are determined with reference to the nature of the study whether it is qualitative or quantitative. They are grouped into appropriate categories and listed in the schedule in the order to make it systematic.

Interview Guide

This is used for non-directive and in-depth interviews. It does not contain a complete list of items on which information has to be elicited from a respondent, it just contains only the broad topics or areas to be covered in the interview. Interview guide serves as a prompter during interview. It aids in focussing attention on salient points relating to the study and in securing comparable data in different interviews by the same or different interviewers.

Rating Scale

This is a recording form used for measuring individual's attitudes, aspirations and other psychological and behavioral aspects, and group behavior in numerical form.

Checklist

It consists of a prepared list of items pertinent to an object or a particular task. The presence or absence of each item may be indicated by checking 'yes' or 'no' or multipoint scale, it may be used as an independent tool or as a part of a schedule/questionnaire.

TECHNIQUE OF DEVELOPING MEASUREMENT TOOLS

Four stages:
1. Concept development
2. Specification of concept dimensions
3. Selection of indicators
4. Formation of index.

SCHEDULE AND QUESTIONNAIRE

Schedules and questionnaires are primary data collection tools contain a set of questions logically related to a problem of a study; both of them are prepared to elicit responses from the respondents of a study; Even though the content, question type, response structure, phrasing of questions, sequence of questions, are same, a schedule is used as a tool for interviewing and questionnaire is used for mailing. That is, the interviewer in a face-to-face interviewing fills a schedule, whereas the respondents themselves fill in a questionnaire.

THE PROCESS OF CONSTRUCTION OF A SCHEDULE AND A QUESTIONNAIRE

The process of construction of a schedule and a questionnaire is not a matter of simply listing questions it is a logical process and consists of progressive developing steps (Fig. 7.1):

PRINCIPLES OF CONSTRUCTION

While following the logical process of questionnaire or schedule construction the researcher should keep the following principles in consideration for the creation of a good and effective tool.

- Clarity of phrased items
- Avoid confusing, difficult to understand, vague phrasing of items
- Provide frame of reference
- Avoid negative phrasing and double negatives

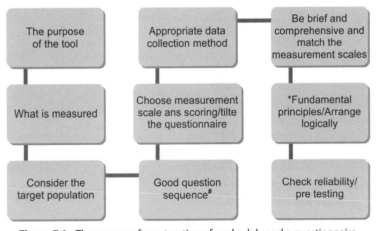

Figure 7.1: The process of construction of a schedule and a questionnaire.

#Good question sequence: 1. Screening items, 2. Warm-up questions, 3. Transitions, 4. Skips, 5. Difficult questions followed by, 6. Classification/demographic details.

*Fundamental principles: 1. Ask only one question at a time, 2. Include simple instructions, 3. Start with non-threatening questions, 4. Use plain language, important questions in the front and avoid loaded questions, 5. Provide space for respondent, 6. Professional look.

- Avoid double barrelled questions
- Minimise risk of bias
- Open ended or close ended items should be decided perfectly
- Allow response space for responders
- Minimise fencing or floating of subjects
- Use matrix form questions to avoid response bias.

DIFFERENCES BETWEEN QUESTIONNAIRES AND SCHEDULES

Differences between questionnaires and schedules is provided in Table 7.6.

Table 7.6: Differences between questionnaires and schedules

Questionnaire	Schedule
▪ Sent through mail	▪ Filled out through the researcher
▪ Cheap and economical	▪ Expensive
▪ More non-response	▪ Non-response is less
▪ Interviewer bias less	▪ Interviewer bias more
▪ Identity of subject not known/no personal contact possible	▪ Identity of subject known/personal contact possible
▪ Time consuming/slow	▪ Well in time
▪ Literates only	▪ Used for illiterates
▪ Large sample size could be covered	▪ Large coverage not possible
▪ Incomplete data-more	▪ Incomplete data-less
▪ Less accuracy of data	▪ More accuracy of data
▪ Observation of subject possible	▪ Observation of subject not possible

DATA PROCESSING OPERATIONS
- Editing of data (field editing, central editing)
- Coding of data
- Classification of data (based on attributes or class interval)
- Tabulation of data (simple or complex).

PROBLEMS ENCOUNTERED IN DATA PROCESSING
- Do not know responses
- Missing forms
- Internal consistency of the data, e.g. Age and date of birth
- Validity checks, e.g. extreme values.

TYPES OF ANALYSIS

The collected data could be analysed in many different ways according to the purpose of the research and its hypotheses. The analysis may be either descriptive or inferential in nature.
- Descriptive analysis

- Inferential analysis
- Univariate analysis
- Bivariate analysis
- Multivariate (regression, manova, canonical and discriminant analysis)
- Causal analysis
- Correlational analysis.

  The aim of this chapter is to give an introduction to the reader briefly about the details of the data collection and not exhaustively. For further information in detail the reader is asked to refer to other print resources.

FURTHER READING

1. Concato J, Shah N, Horwitz RI. Randomized, controlled trials, observational studies, and the hierarchy of research design. N Engl J Med. 2000;342:1887–92.
2. Patricia Pulliam Phillips, Cathy A. Stawarski, Data Collection: Planning for and Collecting All Types of Data. ISBN: 978-0-7879-8718-3;192 pages;January 2008, Pfeiffer.
3. Pawar MS. Data Collecting Methods and Experiences: A Guide for Social Researchers. Sterling Publishers Pvt. 2004 - Social Science - 264 pages.
4. Salkind N. (2010). Encyclopedia of Research Design. Thousand Oaks, CA: SAGE Publications Ltd doi: 10.4135/9781412961288.

Ethics in Research

ETHICS IN RESEARCH

Research that involves human subjects or participants with life raises unique and complex ethical, legal, social and political issues. Research ethics is specifically interested in the analysis of ethical issues that are raised when people are involved as participants of research. **Ethics in research**-need to ensure that no harm occurs to participants as well as no research be carried in the most rightful manner. Interactions with participants of the research may inadvertently harm them in some unintended way. In short, ethics are the rules of right and wrong or norms of conduct those distinguish between acceptable and non-acceptable behavior in our drive through journey of human life. Our learning through formal education, social settings, various life experiences as morals decide norms of decision making in our thoughts and actions. There are many reasons why it is important to adhere to ethical norms in research.

Supposing, imagine a physiotherapist plan to do research on the effects of laser on pressure sores by real observation. And the research team has decided to involve histological or tissue examination of the sample at some defined end points in the research. This may involve biomedical tests wherein the participant need to pay money or sometimes the endpoint may cause deterioration of the condition that the subject is currently enduring or he/she is involved voluntarily in the research as it may provide some new knowledge for the wider benefit of the society. Given these multitude of dimensions in which the research is conducted, the underlying philosophy should be that, the participant, the researcher and the wider society for which this exploration of truth on the subject of interest is being undertaken should be guided by some regulations so that everyone involved benefits without any harm to self or others knowingly or unknowingly. Hence, Ethics need to direct the research in the right direction by promoting the aims of the research, values that are essential to collaborative work, be accountable to support, and a variety of moral and social values. How can you achieve this? We know our moral values are intended not to harm but to help anyone and hence diverse lists of persons should be involved before the conduct of research who can help in controlling possible moral deviations that research journey might take in the conduct of research so that no harm is caused. Here, a committee consisting of people from diverse backgrounds should be involved before embarking on the conduct of research to help the conduct in the right and just way. Generally, the deviations in the research from the intended aim attribute to harms that may arise in the research to the persons involved in the research, which are as follows.

HARMS IN RESEARCH
- Physical harm
- Psychological harm
- Emotional harm
- Financial harm
- Social harm/embarrassment.

Roughly, the general summary of some ethical principles that address various moral codes in the conduct of research are, Honesty, Objectivity, Integrity, Carefulness, Openness, Respect for intellectual property, Confidentiality, Responsible publication, Responsible mentoring, Respect for colleagues, Social responsibility, Non-discrimination, Competence, Legality, Animal care, Human subjects protection. Our direction for research should be governed in every possible way through the ethical principles mentioned above.

ETHICAL PHILOSOPHIES
1. A deontological philosophies focus on the *factors* or *means* used to arrive at an ethical decision (Skinner, Ferrell, and Dubinsky, 1988). It emphasizes moral obligations or commitments that should be binding or necessary for proper conduct based on the defined series of rules than consequences of action.
2. A teleological approach is frequently used in medical research, where the research needs to weigh up the potential harm to

participants versus the harm from them not participating. It emphasizes the consequences that result from an action. In other words, they deal with the moral worth of the behavior as determined totally by the consequences of the behavior.
3. Kantian ethics suggest that "persons should be treated as ends and never purely as means" (Beauchamp and Bowie, 2004).
4. Other ethical perspectives include common morality theory, rights theory, virtue ethics, feminist theories, and ethics of care

ETHICAL ISSUES IN RESEARCH

Ethical issues are exhibit in Figure 8.1.

Voluntary Participation

Historically, during the times of second world war and post era, research was carried out on subjects who were at major physical or psychological disadvantage realising only later that the persons were subjected to persecution or abuse or harm. This means that the participants were not aware of the potential harm or danger they were enduring. This means that participants should be fully informed about the procedures and risks involved while involving themselves in research. The notion of voluntary participation relates to requirement of 'Informed consent' for voluntary participation in the research process understanding the risks involved in the process.

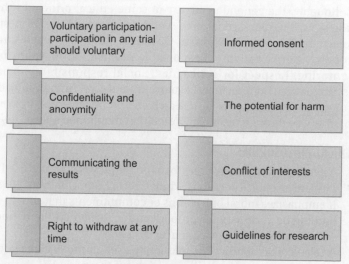

Figure 8.1: Ethical issues.

Confidentiality

- During a survey of teachers, a question asks, "Do you think the administration, especially your principal, is doing a good job?" or when a student course evaluation questionnaire asks, "On a scale of 1 to 5, how fair would you say the professor is?" respondents may well hesitate.

The above scenarios might push the participants to undue harms if they reveal information of what they think as right to them. For example, in the survey of teacher mentioned above, student may be subjected unwarranted harm by a said teacher for revealing truthful information when he/she has acted for a researcher's need. Hence, it is essential that every research activity should guarantee safety of the participants at the time of research proposal itself and should be monitored by the research committee at the conception stage of a research. Some methods to preserve confidentiality of the participants are:

- Only numbers should be used to identify respondents.
- Encryption technology should be used to make information provided over the Internet secure from unauthorized people.

Anonymity

- Where no identifying information is ever recorded to link respondents with their responses. In strict sense this means that the participants remain unknown throughout the conduct of research process. For reasons of changing the result in a desired way, it is essential that participants or the researchers should remain unknown till the end of the study. But strict anonymity is not possible where recordings need to be done multiple times on a subject. However, every possible attempt should be made to keep the anonymity of the participant.

Informed Consent

It is a process of getting the permission from the participants/subjects before the research data collection.

Information sheets should include:

- Who is doing the research?
- Where you are from?
- Why you are doing the research?
- Who the supervisor is?
- How were they selected to participate?

- What do participants need to do and how long it will take?
- Is there any potential for them to be harmed?
- Whether their confidentiality and anonymity will be protected?
- What happens to the data and any report?
- How they will be informed of the results?

Communicating Results

Three broad issues that need to be aware of when completing research project report:
- Plagiarism
- Academic fraud
- Misrepresenting results.

Plagiarism

- Claiming or reproducing someone else's work as your own.
- Avoid Cut and paste work/copy paragraphs.
- Plagiarism is a breach of the student code of conduct and can result in failing.
- "Turnitin" software-automatically checks whether the written matches not only published works, but material in other assignments.

Academic fraud/Misrepresenting results

- Intentional misrepresentation
- Making up data
- Making up results
- Purposefully putting forward conclusions
- Solution: limitation section that identifies unforeseen problems.

Conflicts of Interest

The research may be a good opportunity to gain competitive information, such action would be ethically inappropriate.

Considerations researchers should address in planning of research

- Informed consent
- Gaining access to and acceptance in the research setting
- The nature of ethics in social research generally sources of tension in the ethical debate
- Including non-maleficence, beneficence and human dignity, absolutist and relativist ethics
- Problems and dilemmas confronting the researcher, including matters of privacy, anonymity
- Confidentiality, betrayal and deception

- Ethical problems endemic in particular research methods
- Ethics and evaluative research
- Regulatory ethical frameworks, guidelines and codes of practice for research/personal codes of practice
- Sponsored research
- Responsibilities to the research community.

GUIDELINES FOR RESEARCH

Most universities have also developed guidelines for conducting ethical research (Polonsky, 1998). In Australia, all universities have agreed to have all research comply with one set of ethical guidelines for all types of human intervention. These guidelines were developed by the National Health and Medical Research Council (NHMRC, 2007b) and apply to all types of research. In addition to the guidelines, the NHMRC also produced the Human Research Ethics Handbook, "which is the primary guideline for ethics committees and researchers alike" (NHMRC, 2007a). The very important guidelines and its development have been given in Table 8.1.

Table 8.1: Ethical guidelines for research

Declaration of Helsinki 1964	In 1964, the World Medical Association established this. It provides recommendations to guide researchers in biomedical research involving human subjects. The declaration governs international research ethics and defines rules for "research combined with clinical care" and "non-therapeutic research." The Declaration of Helsinki was revised in 1975, 1983, 1989, and 1996.	▪ Research with humans should be based on the results from laboratory and animal experimentation ▪ Research protocols should be reviewed by an independent committee prior to initiation ▪ Informed consent from research participants is necessary ▪ Research should be conducted by medically/scientifically qualified individuals ▪ Risks should not exceed benefits
National Research Act 1974	The National Research Act created the National Commission for the Protection of Human Subjects of Biomedical and Behavioural Research. The commission drafted the Belmont Report, a foundational document for the ethics of human subjects research in the United States.	▪ Respect for persons—autonomy ▪ Beneficence—no harm ▪ Justice—equal distribution of risks and benefits ▪ Informed consent—voluntary participation ▪ Assessment of risks and benefits—in a systematic manner ▪ Selection of subjects—fair procedures

Contd...

Contd...

Common Rule 1991	In 1981, the Department of Health and Human Services (DHHS) and the Food and Drug Administration (FDA) issued regulations based on the Belmont Report. In 1991, the core DHHS regulations were formally adopted by other departments and agencies that conduct or fund research involving human subjects as the Federal Policy for the Protection of Human Subjects, or the "Common Rule. The 1991 version of the "Federal Policy," as it is known, is widely used.	• Requirements for assuring compliance by research institutions • Requirements for researchers obtaining and documenting informed consent • Requirements for Institutional Review Board (IRB) membership, function, operations, review of research, and record keeping • Additional protections for certain vulnerable research subjects (pregnant women, prisoners, and children)

TEMPLATE FOR INFORMED CONSENT (WHO)

Various online resources are available wherein researchers can search templates for informed consent. Through the following link they can get informed consent templates for different type of studies: //www.who.int/rpc/research_ethics/informed_consent/en/. Please check the screen shots from the computer shown below (Fig. 8.2). The researchers can form an informed consent form in a language which is understood by the participants of the study.

It is not always necessary that a sample templates be followed for every informed consent as the research topic to setting vary. Every researcher or team can decide depending on the need of the research they undertake taking cues from templates and previous informed consent sheets to make it tailored to their purpose. Proforma of sample informed consent is provided below.

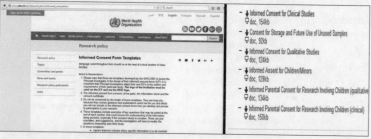

Figure 8.2: Screen shots from the computer for informed consent form templates.

[INSTITUTIONAL LETTERHEAD]

Please do not submit consent forms on the WHO letter head

[Informed Consent Form (ICF): Write the Name the group of individuals for whom this informed consent form is written + **The title of our research project]**

Rewriting to be done

You may provide the following information either as a running paragraph or under headings as shown below.

1. **Name of Principal Investigator**
2. **Name of Organization**
3. **Name of Sponsor**
4. **Name of Proposal and Version**

This Informed Consent Form has two parts:

Part I: Information Sheet

Part II: Certificate of Consent

PART I: Information Sheet

Introduction

Briefly state who you are and explain that you are inviting them to participate in the research you are doing. Inform them that they may talk to anyone they feel comfortable talking with about the research and that they can take time to reflect on whether they want to participate or not. Assure the participant that if they do not understand some of the words or concepts, that you will take time to explain them as you go along and that they can ask questions now or later.

Purpose of the Research

Explain in lay terms why you are doing the research. The language used should be clear rather than confuse. Use local and simplified terms for a disease. There are guides on the internet to help you find substitutes for words which are overly scientific or are professional jargon.

Type of Research Intervention

Briefly state the type of intervention that will be undertaken. This will be expanded upon in the procedures section but it may be helpful and less confusing to the participant if they know from the very beginning.

Participant Selection

State why this participant has been chosen for this research. People often wonder why they have been chosen to participate and may be fearful, confused or concerned.

Voluntary Participation

Indicate clearly that they can choose to participate or not. State, what the alternative - in terms of the treatment offered by the clinic - will be, if they decide not to participate. State, that they will still receive all the services they usually do whether they choose to participate or not. This can be repeated and expanded upon later in the form as well, but it is important to state clearly at the beginning of the form that participation is voluntary so that the other information can be heard in this context.

Procedures and Protocol

Describe or explain the exact procedures that will be followed on a step-by-step basis. Indicate which procedure is routine and which is experimental or research. Participants should know what to expect and what is expected of them. Use active, rather than conditional, language. Write "we will ask you to...." instead of "we would like to ask you...". In this template, this section has been divided into two: firstly, an explanation of unfamiliar procedures and, secondly, a description of process.

A. Unfamiliar Procedures

This section should be included if there may be procedures which are not familiar to the participant. It is important to ensure that the participants understand procedures such as randomization, blinding or placebo. Explain that there are standards/guidelines that will be followed for the treatment of their condition.

B. Description of the Process

Describe to the participant what will happen on a step-by-step basis. It may be helpful to the participant if you use drawings or props to better illustrate the procedures.

Duration

Include a statement about the time commitments of the research for the participant including both the duration of the research and follow-up, if relevant.

Side Effects

Potential participants should be told if there are any known or anticipated side effects and what will happen in the event of a side effect or an unexpected event.

Risks

Explain and describe any possible or anticipated risks. Describe the level of care that will be available in the event that harm does occur, who will provide it, and who will pay for it. A risk can be thought of as being the possibility that harm may occur. Provide enough information about the risks that the participant can make an informed decision.

Benefits

Mention only those activities that will be actual benefits and not those to which they are entitled regardless of participation. Benefits may be divided into benefits to the individual, benefits to the community in which the individual resides, and benefits to society as a whole as a result of finding an answer to the research question.

Reimbursements

State clearly what you will provide the participants with as a result of their participation. WHO does not encourage incentives. However, it recommends that reimbursements for expenses incurred as a result of participation in the research be provided.

Confidentiality

Explain how the research team will maintain the confidentiality of data, especially with respect to the information about the participant which would otherwise be known only to the physician but would now be available to the entire research team. Note that because something out of the ordinary is being done through research, any individual taking part in the research is likely to be more easily identified by members of the community and is therefore more likely to be stigmatized.

Sharing the Results

Where it is relevant, your plan for sharing the information with the participants should be provided. If you have a plan and a timeline for the sharing of information, include the details. You should also inform the participant that the research findings will be shared more broadly, e.g. through publications and conferences.

Right to Refuse or Withdraw

This is a reconfirmation that participation is voluntary and includes the right to withdraw.

Alternatives to Participating

Include this section only if the study involves administration of investigational drugs or use of new therapeutic procedures. It is important to explain and describe the established standard treatment.

Who to Contact

Provide the name and contact information of someone who is involved, informed and accessible (a local person who can actually be contacted). State also that the proposal has been approved and how.

PART II: Certificate of Consent

This section should be written in the first person and have a statement similar to the one in bold below. If the participant is illiterate but gives oral consent, a witness must sign. A researcher or the person going over the informed consent must sign each consent.

I have read the foregoing information, or it has been read to me. I have had the opportunity to ask questions about it and any questions that I have asked have been answered to my satisfaction. I consent voluntarily to participate as a participant in this research.
Print Name of Participant _____

Signature of Participant _____

Date _____

    Day/month/year

If illiterate

A literate witness must sign (if possible, this person should be selected by the participant and should have no connection to the research team). Participants who are illiterate should include their thumb-print as well.

I have witnessed the accurate reading of the consent form to the potential participant, and the individual has had the opportunity to ask questions. I confirm that the individual has given consent freely.

Print name of witness_____ AND Thumb print of participant

Signature of witness _____

Date _____
    Day/month/year

Statement by the researcher/person taking consent
I have accurately read out the information sheet to the potential participant, and to the best of my ability made sure that the participant understands that the following will be done:

1. _____

2. _____

3. _____

I confirm that the participant was given an opportunity to ask questions about the study, and all the questions asked by the participant have been answered correctly and to the best of my ability. I confirm that the individual has not been coerced into giving consent, and the consent has been given freely and voluntarily.

A copy of this ICF has been provided to the participant.
Print Name of Researcher/person taking the consent _____

Signature of Researcher/person taking the consent _____

Date _____

    Day/month/year

FURTHER READING

1. The International Ethical Guidelines for Biomedical Research Involving Human Subjects. http://www.fhi.org/training/fr/Retc/pdf_files/cioms.pdf Last accessed August 8, 2009.
2. Tri-Council Policy Statement: Ethical Conduct for Research Involving Humans, Government Canada. http://www.pre.ethics.gc.ca/english/policystatement/policystatement.cfm Last accessed August 8, 2009.
3. The Nuremberg Code, Research ethics guideline 2005. http://www.hhs.gov/ohrp/references/nurcode.htm Last accessed August 8, 2009.

4. The Declaration of Helsinki, Research ethics guideline. http://www.wma.net/en/30publications/10policies/b3/index.html Last accessed December 22, 2009.
5. The Belmont Report, Research ethics guideline. http://ohsr.od.nih.gov/guidelines/belmont.html Last accessed August 8, 2009.
6. The ICH Harmonized Tripartite Guideline-Guideline for Good Clinical Practice. http://www.gcppl.org.pl/ma_struktura/docs/ich_gcp.pdf Last accessed August 8, 2009.

CHAPTER

9

Research Reporting

RESEARCH REPORTING

Researchers or academicians do engage in research due to many factors or reasons but everyone aims to bring the information that will contribute to the body of knowledge and ultimately benefit patient care in a meaningful way. Adequate reporting of quantitative research results involves careful consideration of the logic and rationale of what has been done by the researcher. Hence researchers need to report the research accurately and appropriately, and then only those who wish to replicate the study can use the information of the reported research. In short, it is a record of the research process till the publication of the findings.

TYPES OF REPORTING RESEARCH

There are various research reporting styles depending on the area where research is undertaken. Two major types of reporting on the findings of a health research are Technical report and Popular report. Figure 9.1 mentions the differences between the two types of research reporting.

1. **Technical Report**
- *Summary:* This gives a brief review of the main findings of the research just in few pages.
- *Nature of the study:* Description of the general objectives of study, formulation of the problem, the operational terms, the hypothesis, the type of study data and analysis are presented in this section.

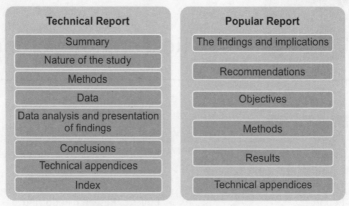

Figure 9.1: Types of reporting research.

- *Methods employed:* Specific methods used in the study and their limitations are presented here. Details of sample design, sample size, sample selection, procedure etc.
- *Data:* Discussion of collected data, their sources, characteristics and limitations.
- *Analysis of data and presentation of findings:* The analysis of data and presentation of the findings of the study with supporting data in the form of tables and charts.
- *Conclusions:* A detailed summary of the findings and the policy implications drawn from the results are explained in this section.
- *Bibliography:* Bibliography of various sources reviewed is mentioned here.
- *Technical appendices:* Appendices be given for all technical matters relating to questionnaire, mathematical derivations, and elaboration on particular technique of analysis.
- *Index:* Index must be prepared and be given at the end of the report.

2. Popular Report

- *The findings and implications:* Emphasis is given on the findings of the study and most/practical implications of these findings.
- *Recommendations:* Recommendations for action on the basis of the findings of the study.
- *Objectives:* A general review of the problem is presented along with the important objectives of the study.

- *Methods employed:* A brief and non-technical description of the methods and techniques used, including a short review of the data on which the study is based, is given in this part of the report.
- *Results:* This section constitutes the main body of the report with liberal use of all sorts of illustrations such as charts, diagrams and graphs.
- *Technical appendices:* More detailed information on methods used, forms, etc. is presented in the form of appendices.

LAYOUT OF REPORTING RESEARCH

A brief layout has been given (Fig. 9.2) for the researcher and the reader to understand the reporting easily.

A standard format in the layout of dissertation or thesis in reporting research with its parts is given below:

1. Preface	2. Main Text or Body	3. End Text/Supplementary
Title Page	Introduction	Instrumentation: Questionnaires, machines, etc.
Original Literary Work Declaration	Literature Review	Appendix: Appendices can be divided into Appendix A, B, C.
Abstract	Methodology	
Acknowledgments	Results	Bibliography
Table of Contents	Discussion	
List of Figures	Conclusion	
List of Tables		
List of Symbols and Abbreviations		
List of Appendices		

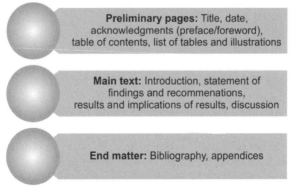

Preliminary pages: Title, date, acknowledgments (preface/foreword), table of contents, list of tables and illustrations

Main text: Introduction, statement of findings and recommenations, results and implications of results, discussion

End matter: Bibliography, appendices

Figure 9.2: Layout of reporting research.

STEPS AND MECHANICS OF WRITING REPORT

Reporting research should be done following the logical steps of the study along with knowledge of accommodating few mechanics of writing to make it legible and easy for the readers or audiences. The following things are to be considered while reporting a research:

- Font size: E.g. 12 or 14; Font size 8 recommended for numbers; font size 15 for title page.
- Theme of font: E.g. Times New Roman
- Page layout: Margins, orientation (Portrait or landscape), size (A3 or A4), Columns (One, two or three), page borders and page color
- Head and foot notes
- Citation style: Vancouver, Harvard, APA style, etc.
- Text alignment: Left, Right, center or Justify
- Punctuation/abbreviation/operational definitions
- Statistics: Descriptive or inferential
- Charts/graphs: Bar chart, pie chart, scatter plot, line graph, etc.
- Rough and fair draft
- Index at the end: Alphabetical index
- Sections must be typed using Times New Roman, font size 12
- A high quality laser or ink-jet printer should be used for the printing.
- The body of the text should be typed with double spacing
- Single-spacing is only permitted in tables, long quotations, footnotes, citation and in the bibliography.
- For mathematical texts, the use of Equation Editor or Latex is advisable.
- The text should have the following margins:
    - Top: 2.0 cm
    - Right: 2.0 cm
    - Left: 4.0 cm
    - Bottom: 2.0 cm
- All page numbers should be printed 1.0 cm from the bottom margin and placed at the right hand side.
- Roman numerals (i, ii, iii etc.) should be used in the Preface section.
- No number is printed on title page.
- Arabic numerals (1, 2, and 3) are used on the pages of the text.
- Footnotes should use a smaller font than the text (font size 8).
- Tables are printed within the body of the text at the centre.

- The label should be placed **above** the table itself.
- If the table occupies more than one page, the continued table on the following page should indicate that it is a continuation: for example: Table 1.1 continued.
- Figure labels are placed at the **bottom** of the figure.
- If the figure or table contains a citation, the source of the reference should be placed at the bottom.
- Recommended to use the End Note software for easy preparation of citation.

SIGNIFICANCE OF REPORT WRITING

To improve or facilitate generalization/external validity of the research. It is important that the authors follow the guidelines so that authors as well as editors, reviewers, readers are able to detail the literature. With electronic formats it has become further easier layering, cross-linking information.

PRINCIPLES OF REPORT WRITING FOR A JOURNAL PUBLICATION

Authors are requested to prepare manuscripts in accordance with "Uniform requirements for Manuscripts submitted to Biomedical Journals" developed by the International Committee of Medical Journal Editors (2016) Available at http://www.icmje.org/icmje-recommendations.pdf

Before Beginning, Answer the Basic Questions

What do I have to say and is it worth saying?
What is the right format for the message that I am going to say?
What might be right for the paper edition of the publication and what for the Web edition?
What is the audience for the message?
What is the right journal for the message?
Another basic rule is to read the instructions to authors by the journal.

Introduction

- Know your audience and for whom you are writing the report
- Tell readers why you wanted to pursue the study
- Clarify what is new in your work
- Follow the best advice/guidelines available on scientific writing for different kind of studies
- Keep the reporting as short as possible

- Make sure that you are aware of earlier studies
- Be sure your readers are convinced of the importance of your question
- Give the study's design but don't give any conclusion in the introduction
- Avoid spinning, difficult and confusing sentences
- The final paragraph of the introduction presents the purpose of the present study
- Instead "we", use an appropriate term such as "people," "humans," or "researchers."

Method Section

- *How the study was designed*
  - Keep the description brief (E.g. Twenty-four consecutive patients, 17 females, (55.73±6 yrs) and 7 males (64.73±8 yrs) with reconstructed ACL tear which is diagnosed by high resolution MRI scanning, who had not previously had physiotherapy input were referred from orthopedic surgeons to take part in the study)
  - Say how randomization was done (random numbers or lottery method)
  - Use names to identify groups or sections of a study (group 1 and 2 or intervention and control group).
- *How the study was carried out*
  - Describe how the participants were recruited and chosen for the study
  - Give reasons for excluding participants
  - Consider mentioning ethical features
  - Give accurate details of materials used
  - Give the exact form of treatment and accessible details of unusual apparatus.
- *How the data were analyzed*
  - Use a *P*-value to disprove the null hypothesis
  - Give an estimate of the power of the study (the likelihood of a false negative the β error)
  - Give the exact tests used for statistical analysis (chosen a priori).

A good methods section can give in depth detail about Participants, Protocol, Assignment, and Masking, Outcome measures, Intervention and Statistical Power and Analysis.

Result Section

- Account for all subjects in the study and double check that the number of subjects is consistent in the abstract, text, tables and figures.
- Be concise in emphasising the important findings and do not repeat information of the tables again in text.
- Avoid using too much of abbreviations.
- Describe the results from each table or figure in a separate paragraph.
- Begin each paragraph with a topic sentence but do not simply repeat the table or figure legend.
- Importantly, do not interpret the results in the results section.

Constructing Tables

- Begin each table on a separate page and number and make it very easy for understanding.
- Do not repeat data abundant in more than one table or figure.
- Provide a concise legend that summarises the content of the table.
- Provide definitions of each abbreviation in the table legend or footnote so that readers no need to refer to the text.
- Clearly mention the number of subjects in each group ('n').
- *P*-value interpretation in a footnote may be appropriate when there are few comparisons. [***Correlation is significant at the 0.05 level (2-tailed).** Correlation is significant at the 0.01 level (2-tailed)**].
- Provide the actual *P*-value, not terms such as '*P* = NS' or '*P* > 0.05'.
- Provide units of measurement, preferably within parentheses after the variable.

Preparing Figures and Illustrations

- Use scientific graphics programmes and avoid yellow and other colors that are difficult to see.
- Clearly labelled axes in black and not less than 0.25 pt.
- Use TIFF or JPEG format for figures.
- Figures should be numbered in the order that they appear in the text.
- Provide a legend for each figure that describes the data.
- The source should be stated clearly in the figure legend.
- Video formats are usually MPEG-4, QuickTime or Windows Media Video.

- Preferred audio formats include WAV or MP3.
- Refer to journal preference for submitting video or audio material (i.e. CD or DVD).

Discussion Section

- Summarise the major findings.
- Discuss possible problems with the methods used.
- Compare for similarities and dissimilarities the study results with previous work.
- Discuss the clinical and scientific implications of the study findings.
- Suggestion can be given for the future research.
- Produce a well fitting conclusion.

Titles, Abstracts and Authors

- Provide a clear indication of what the reader can expect from the paper.
- Indicate why the reader should care to read further.
- List the key methodological details required to understand both how your study addresses the research question and what to expect of the results.
- Describe the results that directly answer the research question (usually including actual values for quantitative studies).
- Summarize the paper with the take home message of greatest importance.
  - Follow the journal's format/length requirements (number of words)
  - Use terms that are likely to be used by colleagues when searching for paper
  - Concentrate on distilling the essence of the paper. And do not promise things that the data cannot provide
  - Catchy title is good, not lengthy
  - Browse articles published by the journal and identify implicit expectations of the journal by journal's author guidelines
  - Write the title and abstract a few different ways to determine which one is the best
  - Read through your paper and highlight the crucial sentences and take opinion from other experts then make corrections based on their feedback.

Contribution Section

Contributors: Name[1], Name[2] ....,
Example (using numbering):
[1] carried out the trial, helped in data analysis and writing of the paper.
[2] was involved in the design, implementation and data analysis
[3] was involved in the execution of the trial, data management and analysis
[4] was involved in the trial execution and data entry, management analysis and quality assurance.
[5] was involved in data management with emphasis on analysis.

Example (using name abbreviation):
Authors' contribution: ATR designed and coordinated the study, performed the statistical analysis and interpretation of the data; MNV revised and reviewed the draft; SNS acquisition and collection of data, Drafted manuscript; DFK acquisition and collection of data.

Acknowledgments Section (According to Vancouver)

At an appropriate place in the article (the title page footnote or an appendix to the text; see the journal's requirements) the author/ researcher should specify

1. Contributions that need acknowledging but do not justify authorship, such as general support by a departmental chair, e.g. The Dean, Director or Principal, etc.
2. Acknowledgments of technical help who helped in drafting the article—a separate paragraph.
3. Acknowledgments of financial and material support—specify the nature of the support.
4. Relationships that may pose a conflict of interest.

GUIDELINES FOR REPORTING RESEARCH

These guidelines can be used for the reporting of designs, data, and analyses of quantitative study designs.

- Researcher may use past tenses to describe the methods used and data collected.
- Provide sufficient information regarding study setting, procedures, and analyses.
- Please compare, contrast and generalize with other studies and settings.
- Report precise frequencies of participants (demographic characteristics or other parameters).

- Describe precisely Sampling, Assignment, and Power.
- Report response rates if survey study.
- Describe exactly the instruments and procedures used to measure values in the study and provide evidence regarding the reliability, validity and consistency of instruments and associated techniques.
- Specify the research design (descriptive, quasi experimental, true experimental, etc.).
- Explain the key variables manipulated.
- Provide proper justification for the specific analyses.
- Avoid repetition of information in tables and graphs that already appeared in the main text.
- Mention "N or n" of participants or cases observed.
- For means comparisons, frequency and correlations, consider graphic techniques.
- Provide effect size estimates and confidence intervals.

ETHICS OF RESEARCH REPORTING

External forces and predetermination of presenting good impact may negatively affect the honesty and accurate reporting of research data. Researchers may wish to present their work in the most favorable way to improve chances of acceptance for publication in reputed journals.

Avoid plagiarism: It is defined as the use of original work, ideas or actual texts created by others, without acknowledging the original source.

Acknowledging the original source: Include the source in the bibliography or include the citation by acknowledging the source in the text.

FURTHER READING

1. Caulfield, RH, et al. The factors considered by editors of plastic surgery journals in evaluating submitted manuscripts. Aesthetic PlastSurg 2008;32(2):353-8.
2. Hamilton CW. How to write and publish scientific papers: scribing information for pharmacists. Am J Hosp Pharm 1992;49(10):2477-84.
3. Roederer M, et al. An integrated approach to research and manuscript development. Am J Health Syst Pharm 2013;70(14):1211-18.
4. Tomaska L. Teaching how to prepare a manuscript by means of rewriting published scientific papers. Genetics 2007;175(1):17-20.

Experimental and Non-experimental Research Designs

TYPES OF RESEARCH METHODS

The research methods can be defined as "a systematic and scientific procedure of data collection, compilation, analysis, interpretation, and implication pertaining to any problem". Methods are pathways of finding answer to a specific research question. For example, a researcher has a question on "What is the best possible treatment for Rotator cuff injury?" The answer may depend on whether the treatment for injury is for male/female, acute/chronic so on and so forth. Every answer that was derived for this question from various research inferences was through various methods or pathways. These pathways are called methods which are processes in deducing answer for a question and they vary depending on the question. Thus, Types of research methods can be classified into several categories according to the nature and purpose of the study and other attributes.

Table 10.1 lists different methods used in various types of research and the strength of answers that were deduced mentioned as level of evidence.

Based on how research is being done Campbell and Stanley (1966) classified research designs into three basic different types:
1. Experimental research design.
2. Quasi experimental research design.
3. Non-experimental research design.

Table 10.1: Types of research methods

Research paradigm	Evidence level of effectiveness	Type	Example	Methods used
Qualitative	Low	Descriptive—Describes a situation or event	Ethnography study, case study	Observations; Interview
Quantitative		Descriptive—Numerical description (means, frequencies)	Survey/cross-sectional	Questionnaires
Quantitative		Correlational/Regression analyses—Relationship between two or more variables	Survey/cross-sectional	Instruments; Questionnaires
Quantitative	High	Quasi experimental—To compare two groups	Non-randomized control trials	Manipulation of variables; Measurement tools
Quantitative		Experimental—To compare two groups	Randomized control trials (RCTs)	Manipulation of variables; Measurement tools
Quantitative		Meta-analysis—Synthesis of results from many studies		Guidelines

EXPERIMENTAL RESEARCH DESIGN

Experimental method is a research method where investigator systematically alters one or more variables in order to determine whether such changes will influence some aspects of behavior. Experimental designs offer the researchers a chance to investigate the *causality of the event* what they are researching due to the high degree of control. Experimental research design contains following components:

- Hypothesis (It is a statement of a particular situation)
- Variables (It is an event or condition, which can have different values)
  - Dependent variable: It is the behavior of the person in the experiment (E.g. Pain)

- Independent variable: It is a condition set by an experimenter (E.g. Lumbar traction).

[Use the terms "independent variable" and "dependent variable" only with experimental research. With non-experimental research use "predictor variable" and "criterion variable."]

- Control (Factors other than the independent variable, which might affect the dependent variable, must be held constant).

One of the key elements of experimental research is *Randomization*. This might help in knowing the real causative change in a research and the assumption is that if there is a real change it is known to have happened by chance. In an experimental research, Subjects are always both randomly sampled and allocated into experimental and control groups. Sometimes the experimenter may focus only on the influence of a single condition, which can be, either present or absent. This method is called Control-group design method. In control group design method one group with the independent variable and the other group without the independent variable. *Thus it is the degree of control that the experimenter can exert over the subject (randomization) and variable (manipulation) are the primary factors in experimental research.*

An extraneous variable is a variable whose presence may compete with the independent variable in explaining the outcome or dependent variable. If an extraneous variable really is the reason for an outcome rather than the independent variable then it is called as *confounding variable* because it has confused or confounded the relationship between the dependent and independent variables.

Control group:
Subjects → No independent variable → outcome measured

Experimental group:
Subjects → Independent variable → outcome measured

TYPES OF EXPERIMENTAL DESIGNS

As there are many types of experimental designs, answers to the following questions may dictate the researcher to what type of experimental design to follow:

- Will there be a control group?
- How many subjects will there be (sample size)?
- Will the subjects be randomly selected (Randomization)?

- Will each group be pretested?
- How will the obtained data be analyzed?
- What factors may affect the internal and external validity?

Experimental design may be classified broadly into Single and Group experimental designs based on the subjects involved. Below mentioned tabular column describes further classification of group design based on the variables involved.

Group experimental design A. Single-variable design B. Factorial design	Single-subject experimental design

GROUP EXPERIMENTAL DESIGN

A. Single-Variable Designs

1. Pre-experimental designs (low degree of control)
   - One-shot case studies
   - One-group pretest-posttest design
   - Static-group comparison design
2. True experimental designs (high degree of control)
   - The posttest-only control group design
   - The pretest-posttest control group design
   - Solomon four-group design
3. Quasi-experimental designs (medium degree of control)
   - Non-equivalent control groups design
   - Time-series design
   - Counterbalanced design
   - Separate-Sample Pretest-Posttest Design
   - Separate Sample Pretest-Posttest Control Group Design.

Examples in various experimental designs are mentioned below. For example, in a study to find if Ice application/Intervention (Independent variable) is effective in controlling spasticity (Dependent variable). This can be done in many different designs and the strength of the design depends as mentioned above on the control of variable.

1. Pre-experimental designs (low degree of control) (Tables 10.2 to 10.4)

Table 10.2: One-shot case study

One group	Intervention /treatment	Posttest measurement
Spastic Cerebral palsy patients (n = 30)	Ice application	Spasticity grade (Ashworth scale)

Table 10.3: One-group pretest- posttest design

One group	Pretest measurement	Intervention/ treatment	Posttest measurement
Spastic Cerebral palsy patients (n = 30)	Spasticity grade (E.g. Ashworth scale)	Ice application	Spasticity grade (E.g. Ashworth scale)

Table10.4: Static-group comparison design

Group 1	Intervention/treatment	Posttest measurement
Spastic Cerebral palsy patients (n = 30)	New ice application method	Spasticity grade (Ashworth scale)
Group 2		
Spastic Cerebral palsy patients (n = 30)	No new intervention/ treatment	Spasticity grade (Ashworth scale)

2. True experimental designs (high degree of control) (Tables 10.5 to 10.7)

In this example, the independent variable is specialized manipulation technique and the dependent variable pain score after treatment.

Table 10.5: The posttest-only control group design

Group	Treatment	Posttest measurement
Randomized group1- experimental group		
Low back pain patients (n = 30)	(E.g. A specialized manipulation technique)	Pain score after treatment
Randomized group 2-control group		
Low back pain patients (n=30)	No treatment	Pain score after treatment

Table 10.6: The pretest-posttest control group design

Group	Pretest measurement	Treatment	Posttest measurement
Randomized group 1-experimental group			
Low back pain patients (n=30)	Pain score before treatment	(E.g. A specialized manipulation technique)	Pain score after treatment
Randomized group 2-control group			
Low back pain patients (n=30)	Pain score before treatment	No treatment	Pain score after treatment

Table 10.7: Solomon four-group design

Group	Pretest measurement	Treatment	Posttest measurement
Randomized group 1-experimental group			
Low back pain patients (n=30)	Pain score before treatment	(E.g. A specialized manipulation technique)	Pain score after treatment
Randomized group 2- control group			
Low back pain patients (n=30)	Pain score before treatment	No treatment	Pain score after treatment
Randomized group 3-experimental group			
Low back pain patients (n=30)	- (no pretest measurement)	(E.g. A specialized manipulation technique)	Pain score after treatment
Randomized group 4- control group			
Low back pain patients (n=30)	- (no pretest measurement)	No treatment	Pain score after treatment

3. Quasi-experimental designs (medium degree of control) (Tables 10.8 to 10.12

In quasi experiments the researcher usually has little control over the 'when' and 'to whom' the treatment (exposure, intervention) is directed. And there is no random assignment of subjects to each group because it is predetermined. As mentioned before, information or inferences generated from quasi experimental studies are relatively low compared to randomized experimental studies.

Non-equivalent control group design is similar to pretest-posttest control group design except that no randomization is required. The groups are generally chosen from clustered units such as classrooms or counselling groups. The major drawback of this design is that since there is no randomization, variables related to history, maturation or testing may interfere with the effect of the treatment.

Table 10.8: Non-equivalent control group design

Non-randomized group 1	Pretest	Experimental treatment	Posttest
Non-randomized group 2	Pretest	No treatment	Posttest

Time-series design is an elaborated version of the one-group pretest-posttest pre-experimental design in the sense that subjects are repeatedly pretested and posttested before and after the treatment rather than being tested once at the beginning and a second time at the end of the treatment.

Table 10.9: Time-series design

One group	Pretest measurement	Intervention/ treatment	Posttest measurement	Repeated measurements
Spastic Cerebral palsy patients (n=30)	Spasticity grade (E.g. Ashworth scale)	Ice application	Spasticity grade (E.g. Ashworth scale)	3rd month
Spastic Cerebral palsy patients (n=30)	Spasticity grade (E.g. Ashworth scale)	Ice application	Spasticity grade (E.g. Ashworth scale)	6th month
Spastic Cerebral palsy patients (n=30)	Spasticity grade (E.g. Ashworth scale)	Ice application	Spasticity grade (E.g. Ashworth scale)	9th month
Spastic Cerebral palsy patients (n=30)	Spasticity grade (E.g. Ashworth scale)	Ice application	Spasticity grade (E.g. Ashworth scale)	12th month

Table 10.10: Counterbalanced design

Time	Session 1		Session 2	
	Group 1	Group 2	Group 1	Group 2
1-4 weeks	Treatment A	Treatment B	Treatment A	Treatment B
	Posttreatment measurement	Posttreatment measurement	Posttreatment measurement	Posttreatment measurement
5-8 weeks	Treatment **B**	Treatment A	Treatment **B**	Treatment A
	Posttreatment measurement	Posttreatment measurement	Posttreatment measurement	Posttreatment measurement

Table 10.11: Separate-sample pretest-posttest design

Group	Pretest measurement	Treatment	Posttest measurement
Randomized group 1			
Low back pain patients (n=30)	No pretest measurement	(E.g. A specialized manipulation technique)	Pain score after treatment
Randomized group 2			
Low back pain patients (n=30)	Pain score before treatment (pretest measurement)	No treatment	No posttest measurement

Table 10.12: Separate sample pretest-posttest control group design

Group	Pretest measurement	Treatment	Posttest measurement
Randomized group 1			
Low back pain patients (n=30)	No pretest measurement	(E.g. A specialised manipulation technique)	Pain score after treatment
Randomized group 2			
Low back pain patients (n=30)	Pain score before treatment (pretest measurement)	No treatment	No posttest measurement
Randomized group 3			
Low back pain patients (n=30)	No pretest measurement	No treatment (control)	Pain score after treatment
Randomized group 4			
Low back pain patients (n=30)	Pain score before treatment (pretest measurement)	No treatment	No posttest measurement

B. Factorial Design

When there are more than two independent variables involved in a study then the design is called factorial design and the variables involved are called factors. Here in the example given, two independent variables or factors involved are specialized manipulation and diabetes. The researcher wants to know whether this treatment has any difference between subjects with low back pain along with diabetes and without diabetes. (Table 10.13).

Table 10.13: Factorial design

Group	Pretest measurement	Treatment	With comorbidity	Posttest measurement
Randomized group 1-experimental group				

Contd...

Contd...

Group	Pretest measurement	Treatment	With comorbidity	Posttest measurement
Low back pain patients (n=30)	Pain score before treatment	(E.g. A specialized manipulation technique A)	(E.g. With diabetes mellitus-YES)	Pain score after treatment
Randomized group 2- control group				
Low back pain patients(n=30)	Pain score before treatment	(E.g. A specialized manipulation technique B)	(E.g. With out diabetes mellitus-NO)	Pain score after treatment
Randomized group 3-experimental group				
Low back pain patients (n=30)	Pain score before treatment	(E.g. a specialized manipulation technique A)	(E.g. With out diabetes mellitus-NO)	Pain score after treatment
Randomized group 4- control group				
Low back pain patients (n=30)	Pain score before treatment	(E.g. A specialized manipulation technique B)	(E.g. With diabetes mellitus-YES)	Pain score after treatment

SINGLE-SUBJECT EXPERIMENTAL DESIGN

Research done with single variable on a single subject. These type of researches may be useful as a starting point before a higher level study. The prime objective of the study is not to study causation and there is no randomization that is involved in otherwise experimental designs. Three common designs in this type are mentioned below.

1. A-B-A withdrawal design: The subject is exposed to a non-treatment condition (A) as well as to a treatment (B) in order to study the difference of behavior within the subject.
2. Multiple-baseline design: These are used when the A-B design is used, and the conditions cannot be reversed.
3. Alternating treatments design: These are used to determine the relative effects of two or more treatments within a single-subject.

THREATS TO EXPERIMENTAL DESIGN

Various types of designs have their own advantages and disadvantages. Validity of the research information is the key attribute through which a claim about the experiment is valued at. This validity claim may be affected by factors within the control environment set for the experiment which called internal validity and which in turn might have an effect on the reliability of the research information. Also, the information from the experiment also need to be ascertained whether it is applicable to the external population and it is essential to analyze in the study about whether any threats affect the validity of the information claim. Table 10.14 lists the factors that may be common threats to internal and external validity in an experimental design.

Table 10.14: Threats to experimental design

Internal validity	External validity
• History threat	• Bias of the experimenter
• Maturation threat	• Hawthorne effect
• Testing threat	• Novelty effect
• Instrumentation threat	• Organismic variable (gender difference)
• Regression threat	• Boredom
• Subject characteristics threat	
• Mortality threat	
• Location threat	
• Implementation threat	
• Data collector characteristics	

STEPS IN EXPERIMENTAL RESEARCH

Issac and Michael (1977) reported seven steps in experimental research as outlined by Van Dalen and Meyer (1966). Figure 10.1 briefs the core steps that are to be followed in any experimental design.

Following these steps is indispensable in making the experimental research information effective one and the purpose for which the type of research design was used.

NON-EXPERIMENTAL DESIGNS (FIG. 10.2)

A design in which the researcher is a passive agent, who observes, measures, and describes a phenomenon as it occurs or exists. In non-experimental research there is no manipulation of the independent variable and there also is no random assignment of participants to groups. In these designs it is only strictly possible to investigate

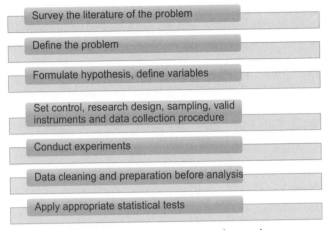

Figure 10.1: Steps in experimental research.

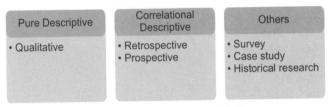

Figure 10.2: Non-experimental design.

associations; the direction of any causal link is purely due to the researcher's interpretation of the results by chance.

Example:

1. Comparative research: Gender of elderly geriatric patients (IV) and performance of balance (DV) [Look for the relationship by comparing the male and female average balance performance levels].

2. Correlational research: Strength of muscles (IV) and fatigue level after performance (DV) [Look for the relationship by calculating the correlation coefficient (r)].

CHARACTERISTICS OF NON-EXPERIMENTAL DESIGN

- No manipulation.
- No establishment of causality.

- A question or hypothesis is proposed.
- A variable, two or more with different level of complexity.
- Gives an overall picture of a phenomenon.

TYPES OF NON-EXPERIMENTAL DESIGN

1. One-Shot (Cross-sectional) Study (Case Study) (Survey)
2. One-Shot Correlational Study
3. One-Group Pretest-Posttest Design
4. Static-Group Comparison Design

DATA COLLECTION METHODS OF NON-EXPERIMENTAL DESIGN

Descriptive

The data collection methods in non-experimental designs are completely tool based. Some forms of tools like phones, recorders, questionnaires, etc. are used to collect the data. The data may be numerical at times or deduced in specific codes. Commonly used data collection methods are listed below.

- Personal interviews
- Telephone interviews
- Questionnaires
- Statistical records
- Observation devices
- Physical measurement
- Psychological measurement
- Reporting
- Rating
- Interview.

Correlational Descriptive

It is a research design where the researchers study the relationship of two or more variables without any intervention. The prime objective of the study is to examine the strength of relationship between variables and determine how change in one variable is correlated with change in another variable.

Two major types of correlational research designs are:

1. Prospective research design
2. Retrospective research design

In prospective design, researcher observes the phenomenon from cause to effect. They are mostly longitudinal but may also be cross-sectional.

In retrospective design, researcher links the present phenomenon with past events. The researcher has a backward movement from effect to identify the cause.

Case Study

The purpose of case study: To analyze the relationships between phenomena. The basis of this method is explanatory in nature, i.e. explain the process with possible relations or associations. Descriptive designs may be used to identify the phenomenon of interest, describe the variables and develop operational definition of variables.

- Explaining
- Describing
- Exploring.

Survey

Survey is a systematic method for gathering information from (a sample of) individuals for the purposes of describing an attribute or many attributes of the larger population in which the individuals are members. The attributes attempt to describe basic characteristics or experiences of large and small populations in our world. The types are:

- Cross-sectional
- Longitudinal
- Trend
- Time cohort
- Panel.

For a survey to succeed, it must minimize the risk of two types of error: poor measurement of cases that are surveyed (*errors of observation*) and omission of cases that should be surveyed (*errors of non-observation*) (Groves, 1989).

CHARACTERISTICS OF A GOOD RESEARCH DESIGN

In summary, whether it is qualitative or quantitative, the characteristics of good research design are:

- Appropriateness to the research problem
- Lack of bias
- Control
- Precision
- Internal validity
- External validity.

FURTHER READING

1. Briner W, Kirwan J. Experimental toxicology: Issues of statistics, experimental design, and replication. Neurotoxicology. 2017;58: 137-142.
2. Gad SC (2001). Statistical approaches to the design of toxicology studies. Curr Protoc Toxicol Chapter 1: Unit1.2.
3. Parab S, Bhalerao S. Study designs. International Journal of Ayurveda Research. 2010;1(2):128-131. doi:10.4103/0974-7788.64406.

Analysis of Variance Study (ANOVA) Designs

ANALYSIS OF VARIANCE (ANOVA)

Analysis of variance (ANOVA) test is used to test the following hypothesis that the means of two or more samples of populations are equal and compared. ANOVA test is developed by statistician and evolutionary biologist called Ronald Fisher. To apply the test Anova, it is necessary that there should be a continuous response variable and at least one categorical factor variable with two or more levels. ANOVAs require data from approximately normally distributed populations with equal variances between factor levels. However, ANOVA procedures work quite well even if the normality assumption has been violated, unless one or more of the distributions are highly skewed or if the variances are quite different. Transformations of the original dataset variables may correct or overlook these violations. The name "analysis of variance" is based on the approach in which the procedure uses variances to determine whether the means are different. The procedure works by comparing the variance between group means versus the variance within groups as a way of determining whether the groups are all part of one larger population or separate populations with different characteristics. The inequality of variance in the model may affect the ANOVA inferential statistical results very slightly, if the model contains only fixed factors and has equal sample sizes however models with random effects and/or unequal sample sizes may seriously and substantially affect the results. When conducting an ANOVA it is always important to calculate the effect size. The effect size reveals the importance of those differences. Effect sizes can be categorized into small, medium or large. Cohen cited, 0.30 as small, 0.30–0.49 as moderate, and 0.50 and greater as large effect size.

DIFFERENT TYPES OF ANOVA

Depending on the number of independent variables (IV) involved in a study, ANOVA can be classified into one or two way ANOVAs. For example in studying the effectiveness of exercises and electrotherapy on the effect over low back pain, it will be a two way ANOVA.

- One way Anova: One fixed factor (levels set by investigator) which can have either an unequal (unbalanced) or equal (balanced) number of observations per treatment.
- Two way Anova: Two fixed factors (levels set by investigator) which can have either an unequal (unbalanced) or equal (balanced) number of observations per treatment.
- Repeated measure Anova: Dependent variable (DV) measured 2 or more times/levels
- Factorial ANOVA-2 or more orthogonal factors
- Multivariate analysis of variance (MANOVA) is used when there is more than one response variable.
- ANCOVA: ANOVA plus 1 or more continuous IVs.

Table 11.1: Types of ANOVA

Number of dependent variables (DV)	Univariate - 1 DV Repeated-measures - 1 DV measured 2 or more times	Multivariate - 2 or more different DVs
Number of independent variables (IV)	One-way - 1 factor	Factorial - 2 or more orthogonal factors
Groups of subjects	Between-subjects - 2 or more groups of subjects, each subject participates in 1 condition	Within-subjects - 1 group of subjects, each subject participates in all conditions
ANOVA plus 1 or more continuous IVs = ANCOVA		

ASSUMPTIONS OF ANOVA

The following are the assumptions in an ANOVA design:
1. Independence (Cases must be independent)
2. Normality
3. Homogeneity of the variances of the residuals (Test that the variance of each condition is roughly equal using Levene's test for between-subjects factors and Fmax for within-subject factors).

Levene's test: If $p > 0.05$, variance is equal enough for ANOVA
Fmax: Less than 4, variance is equal enough for ANOVA.

Test for Equal Variance

Multiple comparisons method and Levene's method.
The F-test and Bartlett's test are accurate only for normally distributed data

4. Sample size should be approximately equal for each group.
5. Samples should not be too small.
6. Sphericity (only for within-subjects designs).

For within-subject factors with more than 2 levels, check for and report sphericity. It is like homogeneity of variance for difference scores between pairs of within-subject factors). Mauchly's Test of Sphericity could be used for checking.

Mauchly's Test of Sphericity: If $p > 0.05$, report the 'Sphericity Assumed' statistics, if not report the Greenhouse- Geisser statistics.

THE ANALYSIS OF VARIANCE (ANOVA) TEST MODELS

In this section each type of ANOVA are described with an example.

1. One way anova

IV (factor)	DV (Continuous variable)
Group 1 (surgery intervention)	ROM of Right knee joint
Group 2 (conventional intervention)	
Group 3 (control)	

Conditions

Three or more samples; Normal data; Unpaired data.
Sample means are compared from groups.

Null Hypothesis

No difference exists between the compared groups, which all belong to the same population.

Alternative Hypothesis

A difference exists between the compared groups and the groups do not come from the same population.

2. Two way anova

IV (Factor)	IV (Factor)	DV (Continuous variable)
Male	Group 1 (Surgery intervention)	
Female	Group 2 (Conventional intervention)	ROM of right knee joint
	Group 3 (Control)	

Conditions

- Three or more samples; Normal data; Unpaired data
- Sample means are compared from groups
- Two independent variables (factors).

Null Hypotheses

- The population means of the first factor are equal
- The population means of the second factor are equal
- There is no interaction between the two factors.

Alternative Hypothesis

- The population means of the first factor are not equal
- The population means of the second factor are not equal
- There is a significant interaction between the two factors.

3. ANCOVA

IV (Factor)	IV (Continuous)	DV (Continuous variable)
Group 1 (Surgery intervention)		
Group 2 (Conventional intervention)	Age in years	ROM of right knee joint
Group 3 (Control)		

Conditions

- Three or more samples; Normal data; Unpaired data
- Sample means are compared from groups
- A covariate is present.

Null Hypothesis

No difference exists between the compared groups, which all belong to the same population on ROM of right knee joint when controlling for age in years.

Alternative Hypothesis

A difference exists between the compared groups and the groups do not come from the same population when controlling for age in years.

4. Repeated measure anova

	Group 1 (Surgery intervention)	Group 2 (Conventional intervention)	Group 3 (Control)
Baseline/before treatment	ROM of right knee joint	ROM of right knee joint	ROM of right knee joint
After 4 weeks	ROM of right knee joint	ROM of right knee joint	ROM of right knee joint
After 8 weeks	ROM of right knee joint	ROM of right knee joint	ROM of right knee joint
After 12 weeks	ROM of right knee joint	ROM of right knee joint	ROM of right knee joint

Conditions

- Three or more samples; Normal data; Unpaired data
- Sample means are compared from groups/level of measurements/ time periods
- The repeated measures design is also known as a within-subject design

Null Hypothesis

- No mean difference exists between the time periods of group 1
- No mean difference exists between the time periods of group 2
- No mean difference exists between the time periods of group 3.

Alternative Hypothesis

- Mean difference exists between the time periods of group 1
- Mean difference exists between the time periods of group 2
- Mean difference exists between the time periods of group 3.

5. Factorial anova

It is used when two or more treatment factors are being compared simultaneously.

Group 1	Group control	Group 2	Group 2 control
Treatment 1 (drug)	Treatment 2 (no drug)	Treatment 1 (drug)	Treatment 2 (no drug)
Treatment A (exercise)	Treatment B (no exercise)	Treatment B (no exercise)	Treatment A (exercise)

Other variations in ANOVA tests such as Post-hoc, Linear model, Greenhouse-Geisser are described in the following sections. Only brief introduction is given and for detailed information the reader is asked to refer also other information sources.

POST-HOC ANALYSIS IN ANOVA

After estimating the F statistic or rejecting null hypothesis using ANOVA in a sample containing various groups, we may also be able to find out which group mean showed variance to reject the null hypothesis. This can be done using post-hoc analysis tests. It is used to determine which mean or group of means is/are significantly different from the others and is only done when ANOVA yields a significant F. There are many different choices depending upon research design and research question (Bonferroni, Duncan's, Scheffé's, Tukey's HSD, etc). Table 11.2 lists three different post-hoc tests and the situations under which they are used and their degree of robustness.

Table 11.2: Post hoc tests

Scheffé test	Bonferroni test	Tukey HSD test
• When sample sizes are unequal • When most conservative test is desired	• Used when less conservative test is desirable, i.e. more powerful • May be used with other types of statistical tests (e.g. multiple t-tests) • When only some pairs of sample means are to be tested	• Sample sizes must be equal but a revised version permits unequal sample sizes (i.e. Tukey-Kramer) • Used when less conservative test is desirable, i.e. more powerful • When all pairs of sample means are to be tested

GENERAL LINEAR MODEL(GLM)

The next statistic variation in ANOVA design is general linear model (GLM). In addition to comparing means of groups just like any ANOVA test does, this statistic is important in analyzing and predicting relationship in a non-normal distribution. It helps in making predictions using continuous variable response and in predicting and understanding behavior of complex biological data. This model is used to determine whether the means of two or more groups differ and include random factors, covariates, or a mix of crossed and nested factors. In this model the calculations are performed using a least squares regression approach to describe the statistical relationship between one or more predictors and a continuous response variable. Predictors can be factors and covariates.

Classes of Models

Based on the ability to predict certain effects the models in GLM are classified into fixed, random and mixed effects models.

Fixed-effects models
Random-effects models
Mixed-effects models

Main effect: It is a difference in population means for a factor (gender) over the levels of all other factors in the design (E.g effect of gender on quality of life score).

Interaction effect: when the effect on one factor is not the same at the levels of another, the effect of one factor depends on the levels of another factor (e.g. gender* type of occupation on quality of life score).

- For a 2-way ANOVA (8 possible outcomes):

Nothing; Main effect of factor A; Main effect of factor B; Both main effects (factor A and factor B); AxB interaction; AxB interaction and main effect of factor A; AxB interaction and main effect of factor B; AxB interaction and both main effects (factors A and B).

GREENHOUSE-GEISSER /HUYND-FELDT STATISTICS IN ANOVA

When Normality assumptions of data was not found or violated for the variables, the use of repeated measure ANOVA of a study can be justified based on the explanations described for correcting for violations of the assumptions of Sphericity. It is a condition where the variances of the differences between all combinations of related groups and levels are not equal which is closely linked to the homogeneity assumption violation and causing the test to become too liberal and increases the Type I error rate. So as to produce a more valid critical F-value and reduce the increase in Type I error rate corrections have been developed by a statistic called epsilon (ε). The value of an epsilon (ε) statistics of 1 indicates that the condition of sphericity is exactly met. If the epsilon statistic decreases below 1 (i.e. $\varepsilon < 1$), indicates a greater violation of sphericity. To estimate the epsilon statistic either the Greenhouse-Geisser or the Huynd-Feldt procedures are used. Then these procedures use their sphericity estimate to correct the degrees of freedom for the F-distribution.

Greenhouse-Geisser Correction

The F-test result is corrected from $F_{(2,10)} = 12.534$, $p = 0.002$ to $F_{(1.277, 6.384)} = 12.534$, $p = 0.009$. The correction has elicited a more accurate significance value. But the p-value has increased to compensate for the fact that the test is too liberal when sphericity is violated.

Huynd-Feldt Correction

The F test result is corrected from $F_{(2,10)} = 12.534$, $p = .002$ to $F_{(1.520, 7.602)} = 12.534$, $p = .005$. Same like the Greenhouse-Geisser correction, this correction also increased the significance value as compensation.

Greenhouse-Geisser vs. Huynd-Feldt Correction

The Greenhouse-Geisser correction tends to underestimate epsilon (ε) when epsilon (ε) is close to 1 (i.e. it is a conservative correction), whilst the Huynd-Feldt correction tends to overestimate epsilon (ε) (i.e. it is a more liberal correction). In general the researers are recommended to use the Greenhouse-Geisser correction, especially if estimated epsilon statistic value is less than 0.75 and use the Huynd-Feldt correction if estimated epsilon statistic value is greater than 0.75. As both corrections produce very similar corrections without much difference, so if the estimated epsilon value is greater than 0.75, the researchers can equally justify using either one of the corrections.

ANOVA RESULT INTERPRETATION AND REPORTING

This section provides a brief overview of the result interpretation in conditions using ANOVA.

Within-Groups Mean Square (Error Mean Square) (MS Within)

This is the average of the variances in each group. It estimates the population variance regardless of whether or not the null hypothesis is true.

Between-Groups Mean Square (MS Between)

This is calculated from the variance between groups. It estimates the population variance, if the null hypothesis is true.

An F-test used should be to compare these two estimates of variance.

Calculated **F Statistic** = variance of the group **means (MS between)/mean** of the within group variances **(MS within)**

Find the F critical Statistic in the F-Table.

- If calculated **F Statistic** is more than F critical Statistic in the table reject the null hypothesis. The F value should always be used along with the p value in deciding whether results are significant enough to reject the null hypothesis. A large f value (one that is bigger than the F critical value found in a table) means something is significant, while a small p value means all the results are significant.
- If the one-way ANOVA is used for the comparison of two groups only, the analysis is exactly and mathematically equivalent to the use of the independent t-test, (the F statistic is exactly the square of the corresponding t statistic).
- If the ANOVA is significant and the null hypothesis is rejected, the only valid inference that can be made is that at least one population mean is different from at least one other population mean.
- The ANOVA does not reveal which population means differ from which others.

Reporting ANOVA: There was statistically significant differences between group means as determined by one-way ANOVA [F (1, 264) = 3.908, p = .049]. If Anova not achieving a statistically significant result does not mean that the researcher should not report group means ± standard deviation also. However, running a post-hoc test is usually not warranted and should not be carried out.

ANOVA

Quality of life score

	Sum of squares	df	Mean square	F	Sig.
Between Groups	.910	1	.910	3.908	.049
Within Groups	61.496	264	.233		
Total	62.406	265			

FURTHER READING

1. Armstrong RA. et al. An introduction to analysis of variance (ANOVA) with special reference to data from clinical experiments in optometry. Ophthalmic and Physiological Optics 2000;20(3): 235-241.
2. Howell DC. Statistical methods for psychology. Duxbury Press,1992.
3. Interpretation and Uses of Medical Statistics by Leslie E Daly and Geoffrey J. Bourke, Blackwell Science, 2000.

4. Madsen, Henrik; Thyregod, Poul. Introduction to General and Generalized Linear Models. Chapman and Hall, 2011.
5. Practical Statistics for Medical Research by Douglas G. Altman, Chapman and Hall, 1991.
6. Shin JH. Application of repeated-measures analysis of variance and hierarchical linear model in nursing research. Nurs Res 2009;58(3): 211-217.
7. Stephens LJ. Advanced Statistics demystified. McGraw-Hill, 2004.
8. Turner JR, Thayer JF. Introduction to analysis of variance: Design, analysis, and interpretation. Thousand Oaks, CA: Sage Publications, 2001.

Pilot Study in Research

PILOT STUDY

Despite the strict guidelines in the conduct of research stresses the importance of doing pilot study as an essential part of any major trial or randomized trials or any research study, it may said that less importance has been attributed to the importance of pilot study. The purpose of this chapter is to give reader key aspect of pilot studies.

The concise Oxford thesaurus defines pilot study as an experimental, exploratory, test, preliminary, trial or try out investigation. Association for Quality Research defines pilot study as, "A small study conducted in advance of a planned project, specifically to test aspects of the research design (such as stimulus material) and to allow necessary adjustment before final commitment to the design. Although not unknown in qualitative research, these are more common in large quantitative studies, since adjustment after the beginning of fieldwork is less possible than in qualitative work." The conduct of pilot study can be equated to this African proverb, "You never test the depth of a river with both feet" similar to the assessing the probable issues that may arise when embarking on a research study.

Definitions

"A trial study carried out before a research design is finalised to assist in defining the research question or to test the feasibility, reliability and validity of the proposed study design."

"A smaller version of a study is carried out before the actual investigation is done. Researchers use information gathered in pilot studies to refine or modify the research methodology for a study and to develop large-scale studies."

"A small study carried out before a large-scale study to try out a procedure or to test a principle."

"A small study often done to assist the preparation of a larger, more comprehensive investigation."

The term 'pilot study' refers to mini versions of a full-scale study (also called 'feasibility' studies). For example: In a survey research it is a specific pre-testing of a particular research instrument such as a questionnaire or interview schedule. Pilot studies are a crucial element for a pre-judgment of a good study design. Conducting a pilot study does not guarantee success in the main study, but it does increase the likelihood of conducting the study in the planned and proposed design. Pilot studies fulfil a range of important functions and can provide valuable insights for other researchers. There is a need for more discussion amongst researchers of both the process and outcomes of pilot studies.

In reality, a pilot study can be used to evaluate if any unforeseen problems may affect the performance during the conduct of research. For example: Pilot study may be helpful in picking up issues involved in the processes involved in a proposed research project like feasibility of recruitment, randomization, retention, assessment procedures, new methods, convincing funding bodies that the proposed research proposal is worth funding and implementation of the novel intervention. In effect, a pilot study is not a hypothesis testing study. Contrary to tradition, a pilot study does not provide a meaningful effect size estimate for planning subsequent studies due to the imprecision inherent in data from small samples. A pilot study is a requisite initial step in exploring a novel intervention or an innovative application of an intervention. Pilot results can inform us on the feasibility and identify modifications needed in the design of a larger, ensuing hypothesis testing study. Investigators should be forthright in stating these objectives of a pilot study. Pilot study is a pivotal part in the conduct of phased drug trials, however, in case of studies involving physiotherapy interventions, where complete blinding is often impossible, it is usually followed that the process is conducted on a small sample initially. Overall thereby increasing total sample size in the research planning is needed and estimation of the sample size can be done based on the effect size.

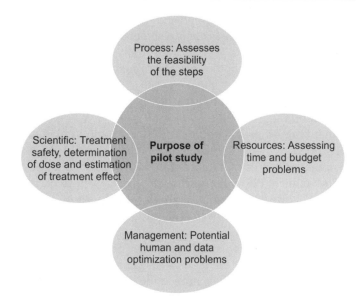

Figure 12.1: Purpose of a pilot study.

PURPOSE OF PILOT STUDY (REASONS FOR CONDUCTING PILOT STUDY)

Van Teijlingen, et al. and van Teijlingen and Hundley have detailed the reasons for performing a pilot study. In general, the rationale for a pilot study can be grouped under several broad classifications—process, resources, management and scientific. (Fig. 12.1).

The lists of reasons for conducting a pilot study are given below:
- Developing and testing adequacy of research instruments
- Assessing the feasibility of a (large/full scale) study/survey
- Designing a research protocol
- Assessing whether the research protocol is realistic and workable
- Establishing whether the sampling frame and technique are effective
- Assessing the likely success of proposed recruitment approaches
- Identifying logistical problems which might occur using proposed methods
- Estimating variability in outcomes to help determining sample size
- Collecting preliminary data
- Determining what resources (finance, staff) are needed for a planned study
- Assessing the proposed data analysis techniques to uncover potential problems

- Developing a research question and research plan
- Training a researcher in as many elements of the research process as possible
- Convincing funding bodies that the research team is competent and knowledgeable
- Convincing funding bodies that the main study is feasible and worth funding
- Convincing other stakeholders that the main study is worth supporting.

For example, researchers want to do research on a question; "Whether clinical Physiotherapists are physically fit to carry their profession?" one can attempt to answer this question in various designs depending on the need and purpose for which they do the research.

If a survey research is planned on the above question, it is essential that the instrument that we plan to use should be a validated one to study the comprehensive nature of the question asked. In case a previous research has been done on this topic, after reviewing from the results of the study, they may plan to make modifications in the instrument so that the shortcomings in the previous attempt can be rectified and betterment in the instrument can be attempted. In effect it is an attempt to negate the shortcomings in the previous instrument based on the results and build a new one which has better accuracy. Now they need to ascertain that the instrument they are going to use would definitely measure what they intent to measure. Then, we subject the tool to study a small group of representative population we intend to study as a piloting process. This would give an insight into the processes that they may encounter at the time of conducting the research. Hence, pilot study is a small model or replica of what they are going to do. They may try to modify the instrument based on the results of the pilot study. Thus piloting helps researchers to refine their search for an answer to the question before embark on the process of journey.

Similarly, before trying to answer the question, the researchers have more number of ways to research the question using various designs. They may try to find the fitness based on certain quantified measure as a baseline and try to establish if the representative population falls into the category so that each of the design would various insights in the topic in question. Hence piloting is a quite essential process in any type of research. Though pilot studies are important part of research, equally pilot studies have limitations that need to be kept in mind which are mentioned in the subsequent parts of the chapter.

THE IMPORTANCE OF A PILOT STUDY

Conducting a pilot study before the research study is very important for the researcher:

To determine the feasibility of the study protocol/procedure

To identify weaknesses of a study

To check and verify the study instrument(s) or tools selection (whether the selected validated tool is appropriate for the target population)

To test the appropriateness of data collection

To test the data collection process – the time taken to complete questionnaire/testing

To judge the subjects' willingness to participate in the study

To test data entry, coding of the items, and appropriateness of statistical tests

To obtain preliminary data for the primary outcome measure (to calculate a required sample size).

PILOT STUDY PROCESS

The processes involved in the conduct of the pilot study are described in Table 12.1.

Table 12.1: Pilot study process

To determine the feasibility of the study protocol	This is to know if the overall conduct of the research study is possible or not? Identify any shortcomings in the steps involved like subject recruitment, retention, refusal, adherence rates of the subjects to the study process, eligibility criteria, instrument effectiveness, data management and analysis, any deviation in terms of proposed funding
Recruitment of subjects	Instructions for randomization are appropriate, issues surrounding, eligibility criteria, difficulty that can be faced with recruitment of the subjects
Testing the measurement instrument	Checking correct operation of equipment, modification in the instrument, intended effect of the equipment, level of intervention is appropriate
Data entry and analysis	Investigators and technicians involved are skilled in procedures, reliability and validity of the data, challenges the study personnel face in the collection and entry of the data

PILOT STUDY EFFECT SIZES AND SAMPLE SIZE DETERMINATION

There has been a tradition of using pilot studies to estimate the sample size necessary for future larger scale hypothesis testing studies. Despite its widespread use, Kraemer et al., 2006 argues that the pilot study results should not be used for sample size determination which is attributable to the inherent impreciseness. The adverse consequences may lead to two types of errors in inferential testing: false positive (Type I error) and false negative results (Type II error).

If a pilot study result size is unduly massive (i.e. a false positive result), future trials are going to be designed with an inadequate variety of participants to provide the applied math power required to discover clinically purposeful effects which would lead to negative trials. If a pilot study result size is very small (i.e. a false negative result), future development of the intervention might be terminated – though the intervention eventually would have well-tried to be effective.

Hence an ideal approach is to determine sample size estimates for a study is based on sufficient statistical power to detect a clinically meaningful treatment effect. However for a new intervention or to study the effect of a new variable or in situations where there are no data from previous studies to inform the process piloting the research study would be the process by which the researcher will be able to proceed further for determining the sample size.

THE MYTHS OF PILOT STUDY

According to Thabane et al. the researchers have few doubts regarding the purpose and usefulness of pilot studies. They claim that a pilot study could be helpful to not only clinicians and trainees, but to anyone who is interested in health research. Their suggestions are given below:

- Can I publish the results of a pilot study?
  - Yes, every attempt should be made to publish.
- Why is it important to publish the results of pilot studies?
  - To provide information about feasibility to the research, to avoid duplication of efforts in assessing feasibility.
- Can I combine data from a pilot with data from the main study?
  - Yes, provided the sampling frame and methodologies are the same.
- Can I combine the results of a pilot with the results of another study or in a meta-analysis?

- Yes, provided the sampling frame and methodologies are the same.
  - No, if the main study is reported and it includes the pilot study.
- Can the results of the pilot study be valid on their own, without existence of the main study?
  - Yes, if the results show that it is not feasible to proceed to the main study or there is insufficient funding.
- Can I apply for funding for a pilot study?
  - Yes. Like any grant, it is important to justify the need for piloting.
- Can I randomize patients in a pilot study?
  - Yes. It is always best for a pilot study to maintain the same design as the main study.
- How can I use the information from a pilot study to estimate the sample size?
  - Use with caution, as results from pilot studies can potentially mislead sample size calculations.
- Can I use the results of a pilot study to treat my patients?
  - Not a good idea!
- What can I do with a failed or bad pilot study?
  - No study is a complete failure; it can always be used as bad example! In fact, it is a success because the researcher avoided wasting time and resources on a study destined for failure!

LIMITATIONS OF PILOT STUDY

A pilot study is not a hypothesis testing study. Quite often, researchers place the importance on statistical significance than feasibility, hence there is a chance that the direction of study gets misinterpreted at the piloting stage itself. Even if the plan of a study is clear, but the objective of conducting a pilot study is not clear say on feasibility or analysis or if it is not based on clear criteria, then the pilot study can be shelved even at the research submission or review phase itself. Hence it is imperative that the pilot study should be approached with clear objective for why it is being done primarily as purpose of checking the feasibility of conducting the study.

It should also be borne in mind that during the piloting of research question the researchers are not evaluating the safety and efficacy of the variables concerned. Pilot study can only examine feasibility of the patient type included in the study. Given the small size of the sample and the objective, the pilot results cannot be generalized.

CONCLUSION

Pilot studies otherwise called as vanguard studies provide a good opportunity to assess the feasibility of the large full scale studies and they can be very informative before a study. For this reason, Pilot studies should be well designed with clear feasibility objectives, clear analytic plans, and explicit criteria for determining success of feasibility. They should be used cautiously for determining treatment effects and variance estimates for power or sample size calculations. Finally, they should be scrutinized the same way as full scale studies, and every attempt should be taken to publish the results in peer-reviewed journals.

FURTHER READING

1. Feeley N, et al. The importance of piloting an RCT intervention. Can J Nurs Res 2009;41(2):85-99.
2. Hertzog MA. Considerations in determining sample size for pilot studies. Res Nurs Health 2008;31(2): 180-191.
3. Thabane L, Ma J, Chu R, Cheng J, Ismaila A, Rios LP, et al. A tutorial on pilot studies: the what, why and how. BMC Medical Research Methodology, 2010, 10, 1. http://doi.org/10.1186/1471-2288-10-1.
4. Van Teijlingen ER, Rennie AM, Hundley V, Graham W. The importance of conducting and reporting pilot studies: the example of the Scottish Births Survey. J Adv Nurs. 2001;34:289-295. doi: 10.1046/j.1365-2648.2001.01757.

Psychometric Properties of Tools

PSYCHOMETRIC PROPERTIES

To put it simple, Psychometrics is a property of an instrument that should accurately and dependably measure what it ought to measure. Numerical measures of psychological phenomenon and attributes are considered as Psychometrics. Though the construct of a Psychometrics can be done in many possible ways, as to the dimensions of attributes they are wide and independent, it is the effectiveness that the instrument measures of what it is purported to measure makes it an effective instrument. It can also be said that psychometrics involves measuring constructs such as knowledge and opinions. Psychometrics is the construction and validation of measurement instruments and assessing if these instruments are reliable and valid forms of measurement. Measurement usually takes place in the form of a questionnaire, and questionnaires must be evaluated extensively before being able to state that they have excellent psychometric properties, meaning a scale is both reliable and valid. (Fig. 13.1).

RELIABILITY

A simple example of reliability can be said thus. Imagine a machine is set to produce soaps in particular dimension and fragrance. Reliability of the machine is that every piece produced by the machine would consistently be the same each time and would match the preset requirements in the production of the soap. Thus, Reliability refers to a measure's ability to capture an individual's true score consistently, i.e. to distinguish accurately one person from another. While a

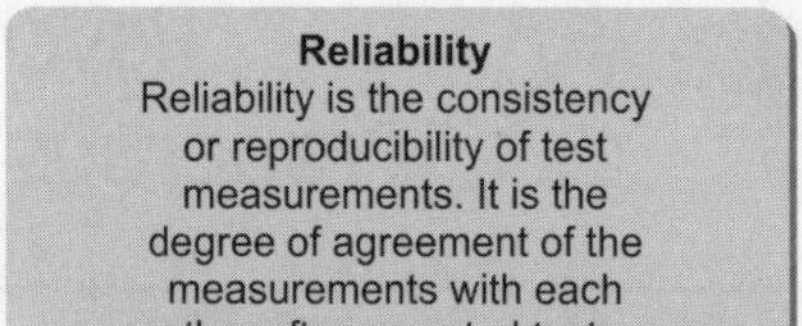

Reliability
Reliability is the consistency or reproducibility of test measurements. It is the degree of agreement of the measurements with each other after repeated tests.

Validity
The degree to which a measure represents what it intends to measure.

Sensitivity
It checks how well a test identifies people who truly have the condition measured by the test.

Specificity
It checks how well the test identifies people who do NOT have the condition being measured.

Figure 13.1: Psychometric properties.

reliable measure will be consistent, consistency can actually be seen as a by-product of reliability, and in a case where we had perfect consistency (everyone scores the same and gets the same score repeatedly), reliability coefficients could not be calculated as there is variance/covariance to give a correlation. The error in analyses is due to individual differences but also the lack of the measure being perfectly reliable.

Criteria of Reliability

Two important criteria based on which it can be said that an instrument is reliable are:

Test-retest reliability
Test components (internal consistency)

Test-retest Reliability

It is the consistency of measurement for individuals over time, e.g. Today and two weeks from now. It is basically reported as Pearson correlation coefficient or intra-class correlation coefficient(r or ICC).

Clinical Importance

- To use an instrument for individual decision-making, it is recommended that an instrument with an ICC > 0.9.
- To use the instrument to measure progress of a large group, an instrument with an ICC > 0.7 is acceptable.

Issues of Test-retest Reliability

The factors that might affect test-retest reliability are:

- Memory: If the correlation between scores is too close in time, in reality there is a chance that correlation might be due to memory of item responses rather than true score captured.
- Chance covariation: Sometimes any two variables will always have a non-zero correlation.
- Reliability is not constant across subsets of a population
  General IQ scores good reliability
  IQ scores for elderly individuals may be less reliable.

Inter-rater Reliability

It determines the variation between two or more raters who measure the same group of subjects.

Intra-rater Reliability

It determines the stability of data recorded by one individual across two or more trials.

Inter-rater/intra-rater Reliability Criteria

Excellent Reliability: ICC > 0.75
Adequate Reliability: ICC 0.40 to < 0.74
Poor Reliability: ICC < 0.40

Internal Consistency

It is the extent to which items in the same instrument all measure the same trait. It is the average correlation among items to assess the reliability of the measure and having more items which correlate with one another will increase the test's reliability. It is typically measured using Cronbach's alpha.

Internal Consistency Criteria

Excellent: Cronbach's alpha > .8
Adequate: Cronbach's alpha < .8 and >.7
Poor: Cronbach's alpha <.7

Cronbach's alpha higher than .9 may indicate redundancy in the scale items.

Replication and Reliability

While reliability implies replicability, assessing reliability does not provide a probability of replication. Note also that statistical significance is not a measure of reliability or replicability. Doing 'exact' replication gives us more confidence in the original finding (should it hold), but may not offer much in the way of generalization.

VALIDITY

Validity refers to the question of whether our measurements are actually hitting on the construct we think what actually they are or whether of concept of interest is correctly captured. While we can obtain specific statistics for reliability (even different types), validity is more of a global assessment based on the evidence available. The researcher can have reliable measurements that are invalid, e.g. The scale which is consistent and able to distinguish from one person to the other could not able to measure what it is intended to measure, e.g. anxiety and depression items are mixed in the scale items.

Criteria of Validity

The different types of validity in an instrument are to be satisfied to make the tool an effective instrument.

Content validity
Criterion validity
Concurrent validity
Predictive validity
Construct-related validity
Convergent validity
Discriminant validity

Content Validity

The items that make up an instrument adequately sample the universe of possible items that compose the construct being measured. Typically assessed by measuring agreement between subject matter experts (SME), although several other techniques (Delphi method) can also be used. Does the question or items mentioned in the instrument cover all the domains of a given construct?

For example, Disability = Pain, ROM, Muscle power, deformities, ADL constraints etc. An example is given below on how content validity of a translated Gujarati language version of a questionnaire is done. And within content validity, three important concepts of equivalence, relevance and representativeness are to be analyzed.

1. **Content equivalence was assessed under two headings:**
   i. Are the words in the translated Gujarati version presented fluently and correctly as in the original version? For this answers from 30 expert panel members fall between 'mostly agree' to 'strongly agree' on a 5 or 7-point Likert scale.
   ii. Do the words and phrase in the translated Gujarati version have the same semantic meaning compared with the original version? For this answers from 30 expert panel members fall between 'mostly agree' to 'strongly agree' on a 5 or 7-point Likert scale.

3. **Content relevance** is assessed by asking: How the Gujarati statement is relevant to assessing disability in back pain patients? For this answers from 30 expert panel members fall between 'mostly agree' to 'strongly agree'.

4. **Content representativeness** was assessed by asking "How well the content of the scale is representing the entire domain of assessing the disability of patients with back pain?" For this answers from 30 expert panel members falls between 'mostly agree' to 'strongly agree' on a 5 or 7-point Likert scale.

Criterion Validity

It is the degree to which the measure correlates with various outcomes. Or in other words whether the tool that the researcher has developed satisfies the entire criterion mentioned in the other standard tool and the outcomes for the variable.

For example, Does some new neck disability measure correlate with the disabilities of the arm, shoulder and hand (DASH) scale.

Concurrent Validity

Establishes validity when two measures are taken at relatively the same time, often indicates that the test could be used instead of a gold standard. When there is consistent relationship between the scores from two measurement procedures – one that the researcher has developed and the other which is kept standard until now (Criterion is in the present).

Predictive Validity

It indicates that the ability of the outcomes of an instrument to predict a future state or outcome. This is possible only when the tool consists of the relevant contents in the construct related to the gold standard (Criterion is in the future).

Convergent Validity

Convergent validity refers to the degree to which two measures from two tools demonstrate similar results, that is the degree to which these two assessments converge provides evidence of the new measure's validity. Convergent validity is a measure of the construct validity of the instrument (Correlates well with other measures of the construct), e.g. Pain scale correlates well with other pain scales.

Discriminant Validity

Discriminant validity is the degree to which two or more measures, assessing theoretically different constructs, demonstrate a difference in outcomes. High correlations between measures (greater than 0.90) indicate the measures are assessing the same domain and may be redundant, e.g. Depression scale *Vs* Stress scale.

Criteria for Predictive Validity, Concurrent Validity, Convergent Validity and Discriminant Validity

The below mentioned statistic values gives the description of various validities in terms of its qualitative significance.
Excellent: Correlation coefficient > 0.6
Adequate: Correlation coefficient 0.31 – 0.59
Poor: Correlation coefficient < 0.30.

Receiver Operating Characteristic (ROC) Analysis - Area Under the Curve

Excellent: > 0.9
Adequate: 0.7 – 0.89
Poor: < 0.7

Construct-related Validity

It is an actual measure of the construct of interest and the ability of an instrument to measure an abstract concept and the degree to which the instrument reflects the theoretical components of it. It includes convergent and discriminant validity which informs about the quality of an instrument as a whole. Construct validity includes

Content, Construct and Criteria related validity which are details about components of the instrument.

SENSITIVITY AND SPECIFICITY

Sensitivity and specificity are also measures of validity for a diagnostic test where the two level (dichotomous) situations of results are met as positive or negative.

Sensitivity

Sensitivity is the proportion of true positives identified by the test. For example, If a test is developed and said that it perfectly identifies all the patients suffering from supraspinatus tendinitis, then it is called a highly sensitive test.

Specificity

Specificity is the proportion of true negatives identified by the test. Similarly when a test developed can also identify all the patients not suffering from supraspinatus tendinitis, and then it is called a highly specific test.

	Disease status	
Test result	**Yes**	**No**
Positive	True positive (TP)	False positive (FP)
Negative	False negative (FN)	True Negative (TN)

Sensitivity = TP/(TP + FN)
Specificity = TN/(FP + TN)
Prevalence = (TP + FN)/(TP + FN + FP + TN)
Positive Predictive Value = TP/(TP + FP)
Negative Predictive Value = TN/(FN + TN)
Positive Likelihood = SENS/(1-SPEC)
Negative Likelihood = (1-SFNS)/SPFC
Overall Accuracy = (TP + TN)/(TP + FP + FN + TN)

A high level of sensitivity and specificity is desirable for a good testing tool or measure. But often there is chance of anyone is high the other one is low. A highly sensitive test, even not very specific 'rules out' a disease condition, i.e. a highly sensitive test is negative rules out a disease (SnNOUT).Similarly a highly specific test, even if not highly sensitive 'rules in' disease condition, i.e. a highly specific test is positive rules in a disease (SpPIN).

OTHER MEASURES OF PSYCHOMETRICS

Floor Effects and Ceiling

Floor Effects

Floor effects occur when a measure's lowest score is unable to assess a patient's level of ability. For example, a psychometric tool or measure that assesses patient's satisfaction for treatment may not be sensitive enough to assess low or intermittent levels of satisfaction. The verbal description of a tool based on its effectiveness in a given sample is mentioned below:

Excellent: No floor effects

Adequate: Floor effects < 20% of lower scores in the sample

Poor: Floor effects for > 20% of lower scores in the sample

OR

Skewness > +1

Ceiling Effects

Ceiling effects occur when a measure's highest score is unable to assess a patient's level of ability. For example, a patient's pre-rehab score may be in-range at the initial evaluation, but the patient's ability exceeds the measure's highest score over time. Therefore, a psychometric tool is unable to accurately assess progress as the patient improves, when there is real improvement. The verbal description of a tool is mentioned below based on its effectiveness in a chosen sample.

Excellent: No ceiling effects

Adequate: Ceiling effects < 20% of high scores in the sample

Poor: Ceiling effects > 20% of high scores in the sample

OR

Skewness < –1

Standard Error of Measurement

The standard error of measurement (SEM) is a reliability measure that assesses response stability. The SEM estimates the standard error in a set of repeated scores. The SEM is the amount of error that is considered as measurement error. In other words SEM is the estimate from repeated scores on a same person with same instrument to find out the true score. However true score can never be found as no construct in a tool can provide perfect reflection of true score.

The equation used to calculate the SEM:

SEM = Standard deviation from the 1st test × [square root of (1-ICC)]

Minimal Detectable Change (MDC)

The MDC is the minimum amount of change in a patient's score that ensures the change isn't the result of measurement error.
The equation used to calculate the MDC:

$$\text{MDC} = 1.96 \times \text{SEM} \times \text{square root of } 2$$

Minimal Clinically Important Difference (MCID)

MCID represents the smallest amount of change in an outcome that might be considered important by the patient or clinician. The MCID is a published value of change in an instrument that indicates the minimum amount of change required for your patient to feel a difference in the variable you are measuring. It is calculated by various different ways.

Using the one-half standard deviation of outcome
At least one standard error of measurement
An effect size cut off point

PRINCIPLES OF TESTING OR TEST CONSTRUCTION

The following verbal description lists the minimum criteria definitions for developing and testing a psychometric tool.

Reliability: It means consistency or accuracy of the test. Studies on reliability tell us whether the test scores are self-consistent and show how good is the test. Reliable tests, whatever they measure, yield comparable scores upon repeated administration. For accurate predictions high reliability is essential.

Validity: It means purpose or truthfulness of the test. Studies of validity tell us how the tests measure what they are supposed to measure and how well they predict according to an acceptable criterion

Standardization: Standardized tests are tests, which have been carefully constructed by experts after try out analysis and revision. They have explicit instructions for standard administration and tables of norms for score interpretation

Objectivity: In a test, measurement, administration, or procedure, scoring and interpretation of scores should be objective irrespective of the researcher.

Interpretation norms: It is an average, common or standard performance under experimental conditions. The norms are in the form of age, grade percentile rank and standard score. These norms should be meaningful and accurate.

Simplicity: A test should be simple in terms of procedure for administration, collection, scoring and interpretation of data. Further, simple language should be used in the psychological tests.

Interpretation economy: There should be economy in terms of the duration for administering the test and the expenses involved in testing.

Definitions of measurement properties of a health-related patient-reported outcome measure (Mokkink et al., 2010)

Reliability: The degree to which the measurement is free from measurement error.

Reliability (extended definition): The extent to which scores for patients who have not changed are the same for repeated measurement under several conditions. For example, using different sets of items from the same HR-PROs (internal consistency), over time (test-retest) by different persons on the same occasion (interrater) or by the same persons (i.e. raters or responders) on different occasions (intrarater).

Internal consistency: The degree of the interrelatedness among the items.

Reliability: The proportion of the total variance in the measurements which is because of "true"a differences among patients.

Measurement error: The systematic and random error of a patient's score that is not attributed to true changes in the construct to be measured.

Validity: The degree to which an health-related patient-reported outcomes (HR-PRO) instrument measures the construct(s) it purports to measure.

Content validity: The degree to which the content of an HR-PRO instrument is an adequate reflection of the construct to be measured

Face validity: The degree to which (the items of) an HR-PRO instrument indeed looks as though they are an adequate reflection of the construct to be measured.

Construct validity: The degree to which the scores of an HR-PRO instrument are consistent with hypotheses (for instance with regard to internal relationships, relationships to scores of other instruments, or differences between relevant groups) based on the assumption that the HR-PRO instrument validly measures the construct to be measured.

Structural validity: The degree to which the scores of an HR-PRO instrument are an adequate reflection of the dimensionality of the construct to be measured.

Hypotheses testing: Idem construct validity.

Cross-cultural validity: The degree to which the performance of the items on a translated or culturally adapted HR-PRO instrument are an adequate reflection of the performance of the items of the original version of the HR-PRO instrument.

Criterion validity: The degree to which the scores of an HR-PRO instrument are an adequate reflection of a "gold standard."

Responsiveness: The ability of an HR-PRO instrument to detect change over time in the construct to be measured.

Interpretability (an important characteristic of a measurement instrument): The degree to which one can assign qualitative meaning—that is, clinical or commonly understood connotations—to an instrument's quantitative scores or change in scores.

CROSS-CULTURAL ADAPTATIONS

Translating a questionnaire instead of creating a questionnaire allows comparisons of different populations, permits researchers to examine functional status across a broad spectrum of people, and permits the exchange of information across cultural and linguistic barriers. It is now widely recognized that questionnaires intended for use across cultures must not only be translated well linguistically but also adapted culturally in order to maintain the content validity of the instrument. The main aim of cross-cultural adaptation (CCA) of a questionnaire is to achieve equivalence between the original and adapted questionnaire using reliable CCA methods. Several methods are available for CCA of questionnaires. According to experts only, most would achieve comparable results, and choosing one is a matter of preference and logistic. Even though more than 31 identified guidelines are found there seem to be no consensus in CCA methods. Most methods included use of committees, focus groups, and back translations. Evidence for the best methods is lacking, although clues indicate that back translation may not be mandatory. More evidence is needed to support recommendations. Adaptation and validation of a questionnaire are two different processes that should be distinguished and undertaken with care. A brief listing of the stages involved in CCA is mentioned below.

Guidelines for the Process of Cross-cultural Adaptation of Self-reported Measures (Table 13.1)

1. Beaton DE, Bombardier C, Guillemin F, Ferraz MB. Guidelines for the process of cross-cultural adaptation of self-report measures. Spine. 2000;25(24):3186-91.
2. Lenderking WR. Comments on the ISPOR Task Force Report on Translation and Adaptation of Outcomes Measures: guidelines and the need for more research. Value in health : the journal of the International Society for Pharmacoeconomics and Outcomes Research. 2005;8(2):92-3.
3. Swaine-Verdier A, Doward LC, Hagell P, Thorsen H, McKenna SP. Adapting quality of life instruments. Value in health : the journal of the International Society for Pharmacoeconomics and Outcomes Research. 2004;7 Suppl 1:S27-30.

Table 13.1: Stages of CCA guidelines (Beaton et al, 2000)

Stages	Process	Outcome
1	Translation	T1- T2 (forward in outcome language)
2	Synthesis	T12 (a version ready for backward translation in outcome language)
3	Back translation	BT1-BT2 (backward translations into English)
4	Expert committee review	Review the methodologists, translators, developer or provider
5	Pretesting	Test with n = (30–40) sample
6	Appraisal by developers or committee	Final version

FURTHER READING

1. Alanazi F, et al. Translation and Validation of the Arabic Version of the Fear-Avoidance Beliefs Questionnaire in Patients With Low Back Pain. Spine (Phila Pa 1976) 2017;42(7): E411-e416.
2. Cronbach LJ. Essentials of psychological testing, 5th ed. New York: Harper Collins; 1990.
3. Mokkink LB, Terwee CB, Patrick DL, Alonso J, Stratford PW, Knol DL, et al. The COSMIN study reached international consensus on taxonomy, terminology, and definitions of measurement properties for health-related patient-reported outcomes. J Clin Epidemiol. 2010;63:737–45.
4. Montazeri A, Goshtasebi A, Vahdaninia M, Gandek B. The short form health survey (SF-36): Translation and validation study of the Iranian version. Qual Life Res. 2005;14:875–82.
5. Ornetti, P, et al. Cross-cultural adaptation and validation of the French version of the Knee injury and Osteoarthritis Outcome Score (KOOS) in knee osteoarthritis patients. Osteoarthritis Cartilage 2008;16(4): 423-8.
6. Vernon H, Mior S. The neck disability index: a study of reliability and validity. J Manipulat Physiol Ther. 1991;14:409–15.

CHAPTER

14

Qualitative Research

QUALITATIVE RESEARCH

Qualitative research is a type of non-quantitative analysis or analysis of data that are not numerical quantification. Qualitative research is collecting, analyzing and interpreting data by observing what people do and say in their life. Qualitative research refers to the meanings, definitions, characteristics, symbols, metaphors, and description of things following by analyzing it towards a common meaning. Qualitative research is much more subjective and uses very different methods of collecting information, mainly individual, in-depth interviews and focus groups.

The nature of this type of research is exploratory and open ended. Small numbers of people are interviewed in depth and/or a relatively small number of focus groups are conducted. Qualitative research can be further classified into the following types:

PHENOMENOLOGY

It is a form of research in which the researcher attempts to understand how one or more individuals experience a phenomenon. For example, The researcher might interview 10 amputees who lost their limbs in a war. This type of research is used to study areas in which there is little knowledge available (Donalek, 2004). In phenomenological research, respondents are asked to describe their experiences as they perceive them. They may write about their experiences, but information is generally obtained through interviews. Phenomenological research would ask a question such as, "What is it like for a mother to live with a teenage child who is dying of cancer?"

Phenomenological Study

For example:

1. Kanagasabai PS, Mirfin-Veitch B, Hale LA, Mulligan H. A Child-centered Method of Interviewing Children with Movement Impairments. Phys Occup Ther Pediatr. 2017 Sep 22:1-14. doi: 10.1080/01942638.2017.1365322. [Epub ahead of print]PMID: 28937834.

2. Hyland G, Hay-Smith J, Treharne G. Women's experiences of doing long-term pelvic floor muscle exercises for the treatment of pelvic organ prolapse symptoms.Int Urogynecol J. 2014;25(2):265-71. doi: 10.1007/s00192-013-2202-z. Epub 2013 Aug 17.PMID: 23955582

ETHNOGRAPHY

This type of research focuses on describing the culture of a group of people. A culture is the shared attributes, values, norms, practices, language, and material things of a group of people. For example: The researcher might decide to go and live with the tribal in Andaman island and study the culture and their educational practices. Cameron (1990) wrote that ethnography means "learning from people". The researcher frequently lives with the people and becomes a part of their culture. Data are generally collected through participant observation and interviews. The aim of ethnography researcher is to learn from members of the cultural group. Ethnography has been the principal method used by anthropologists to study people all over the world. The outcome of this research is mostly story- telling and it is unable to generalize the research findings. Ethnographers study how people live and how they communicate with each other.

Ethnographic Study

For example:

1. Thomson D. An ethnographic study of physiotherapists' perceptions of their interactions with patients on a chronic pain unit. Physiother Theory Pract. 2008;24(6):408-22. doi: 10.1080/09593980802511805.PMID: 19117232.

2. Majumdar SS, Luccisano M, Evans C. Perceptions of physiotherapy best practice in total knee arthroplasty in hospital outpatient settings. Physiother Can. 2011;63(2):234-41. doi: 10.3138/ptc.2010-09. Epub 2011 Apr 13.PMID: 22379264

CASE STUDY

It is a form of qualitative research that is focused on providing a detailed account of one or more cases. For example: We may study a classroom that was given a new curriculum for technology use. A case study or case report may be considered as quantitative or qualitative research depending on the purpose of the study and the design chosen by the researcher. As is true of other types of qualitative studies, for a case study to be considered as a qualitative study, the researcher must be interested in the meaning of experiences to the subjects themselves, rather than in generalizing results to other groups of people. Case studies are not used to test hypotheses, but hypotheses may be generated from case studies (Younger, 1985). Data may be collected in case studies through various means such as questionnaires, interviews, observations, or written accounts by the subjects. Content analysis is used in evaluating the data from case studies. Content analysis involves the examination of communication messages. The researcher searches for patterns and themes.

Case Study

For example:
1. Jang SH, Lee HD. Delayed recovery of the affected finger extensors at chronic stage in a stroke patient: A case report. Medicine. 2017;96(43):e8023.
2. Do J, Jeon J, Kim W. The effects of bandaging with an additional pad and taping on secondary arm lymph edema in a patient after mastectomy. Journal of Physical Therapy Science. 2017; 29(7):1272-5

GROUNDED THEORY

It is an inductive type of research, based or grounded in the observations of data from which it was developed; it uses a variety of data sources, including quantitative data, review of records, interviews, observation and surveys. Grounded theory is a qualitative research approach developed by two sociologists, Glaser and Strauss (1967).The grounded theory method uses both an inductive and a deductive approach to theory development. According to Field and Morse (1985), "constructs and concepts are grounded in the data and hypotheses are tested as they arise from the research. According to Jacelon and O'Dell (2005), grounded theory is an excellent method for understanding the processes through which patients learn to manage new or chronic health problems. Each individual may manage the health problem in a different way. For example, A nurse researcher might be interested in how young women deal with premenstrual syndrome (PMS).The researcher looks for certain subjects who will be able to shed new light on the phenomenon being studied. Diversity rather than similarity is sought in the people that are sampled. Data collection primarily consists of participant observation and interviews, and data are recorded through handwritten notes and tape recordings. Grounded theory is more concerned with the generation rather than the testing of hypotheses.

Grounded Theory

For example:

1. Timothy EK, Graham FP, Levack WM. Transitions in the Embodied Experience After Stroke: Grounded Theory Study. Phys Ther. 2016; 96(10):1565-1575. Epub 2016 Apr 21. PMID: 27103225.

2. Thomson OP, Petty NJ, Moore AP. Clinical decision-making and therapeutic approaches in osteopathy - a qualitative grounded theory study. Man Ther. 2014;19(1):44-51. doi: 10.1016/j.math.2013.07.008. Epub 2013 Aug 7.PMID: 23932101

HISTORICAL RESEARCH

It allows one to discuss past and present events in the context of the present condition, and allows one to reflect and provide possible answers to current issues and problems. For example, The lending pattern of business in the 19th century Leininger (1985) wrote, "Without a past, there is no meaning to the present, nor can we develop a sense of ourselves as individuals and as members of groups". The data for historical research are usually found in documents or in relics and artifacts. Documents may include a wide range of printed material. Relics and artifacts are items of physical evidence. The sources of historical data are frequently referred to as primary and secondary sources. Examples of primary sources: oral histories, written records, diaries, eyewitnesses, pictorial sources, and physical evidence.

Historical Study

For example:

1. Yang XY, Ma YX, Tian SS, Gao SZ. Zhongguo Zhen Jiu. Ancient clinical application of massage therapy on navel. 2014;34(7):719-20. Chinese. PMID: 2523367.

2. Silver JR, Weiner MF. Electrical treatment of spinal cord injuries in the 18th and 19th centuries. J Med Biogr. 2013;21(2):75-84. doi: 10.1258/jmb.2012.012014.PMID: 24585746

ACTION RESEARCH STUDY

Action research is a type of qualitative research that seeks action to improve practice and study the effects of the action that was taken (Streubert and Carpenter, 2002). Solutions are sought to practice problems in one particular hospital or health care setting. For any action research the following seven steps forms a cyclical path till a convincing answer is reached. The seven steps are:

1. Selecting a focus
2. Clarifying theories
3. Identifying research questions
4. Collecting data
5. Analyzing data
6. Reporting results
7. Taking informed action.

However, there is no goal of trying to generalize the findings of the study, as is the case in quantitative research studies. In action research, the implementation of solutions occurs as an actual part of the research process. There is no delay in implementation of the solutions. Kurt Lewin (1946) was influential in spreading action research.

Action Research Study

For example:
1. Action research as a method for changing patient education practice in a clinical diabetes setting; Jane R Voigt Ulla M Hansen Mette GlindorfRiePoulsen Ingrid Willaing Action Research, vol. 12, 3: pp. 315-336. First Published May 8, 2014.
2. An action research project to explore, implement and evaluate the use of rehabilitation guidelines for physiotherapy in the critically ill, Elliott, S. Physiotherapy, Volume 101, e356 - e357;DOI: http://dx.doi.org/10.1016/j.physio.2015.03.569.

TYPES OF INFORMATION COLLECTED IN QUALITATIVE RESEARCH

- Observations
- Interviews
- Documents
- Audio-Visual Materials

ANALYSIS OF THE DATA IN QUALITATIVE RESEARCH CODING STEPS

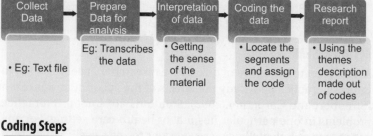

Collect Data → Prepare Data for analysis → Interpretation of data → Coding the data → Research report

- Eg: Text file
- Eg: Transcribes the data
- Getting the sense of the material
- Locate the segments and assign the code
- Using the themes description made out of codes

Coding Steps

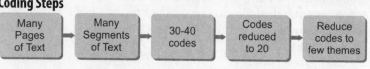

Many Pages of Text → Many Segments of Text → 30-40 codes → Codes reduced to 20 → Reduce codes to few themes

Computer Programs available for analysis of data:

Atlas.ti- http://www.atlasti.de/index.html
N6 -http://www.qsrinternational.com/
NVivo- http://www.qsrinternational.com/
Maxqda- http://www.maxqda.com

QUANTITATIVE *VS* QUALITATIVE RESEARCH METHODS

Quantitative and qualitative research methods differ primarily in their analytical objectives, the types of research problems intended to solve, flexibility of the study design, the types of data collection instruments used and the forms of data collected for analysis. One advantage of qualitative methods in exploratory research is that use of open-ended questions and probing gives participants the opportunity to respond in their own words, rather than forcing them to choose from fixed responses, as quantitative methods do. Open-ended questions have the ability to evoke responses that are:

- Meaningful and culturally salient to the participant
- Unanticipated by the researcher
- Rich and explanatory in nature.

Another advantage of qualitative methods is that they allow the researcher the flexibility to probe initial participant responses – that is, to ask why or how. The researcher must listen carefully to what participants say, engage with them according to their individual personalities and styles, and use "probes" to encourage them to elaborate on their answers. Table 14.1 compares the major differences between quantitative and qualitative research methods.

Table 14.1: Quantitative *Vs* qualitative research methods

Characteristics	Quantitative	Qualitative
Framework	To confirm hypothesis	To explore
Objectives	To quantify, analyse and predict	To describe
Sampling	Rigid	Purposive
Data collection tools	Clinical measurements, survey instruments	In-depth interviews, focus group discussions, obtrusive and unobtrusive observation
Data	Numerical	Textual
Design	Stable	Flexible and iterative
Research question	Focused	Open and flexible
Analysis	Statistical	Thematic
Presentation	By tables and graphs	Theme illustrations

FURTHER READING

1. Bryman A. Quantitative and qualitative research: further reflections on their integration. In: Brannen J, editor. Mixing methods: qualitative and quantitative research. Aldershot: Avebury; 1992.
2. Denzin NK, Lincoln YS. Handbook of Qualitative Research, 2nd edition. London: Sage 2000.
3. Jimmie Manning, Adrianne Kunkei, Researching Interpersonal Relationships: Qualitative Methods, Studies, and Analysis, Sage Publishers, 2014.
4. Neuman, William Lawrence. Social research methods: Quantitative and qualitative approaches. Allyn and Bacon, 2005.
5. Qualitative Inquiry and Research Design: Choosing Among Five Approaches. By Creswell, 2013, 3rd edition
6. Qualitative Research and Evaluation Methods, Michael Quinn Patton, 2002.
7. Silverman D. Doing Qualitative Research: A Practical Handbook: SAGE Publications; 2005.

Survey Research

SURVEY

Survey is a research design in which the collection of information is done from a sample of individuals through their responses to question. It is an important area of applied social research. It is a systematic way of gathering information from a sample of individuals for the purpose of describing the attributes of the larger population. Surveys are mainly conducted for the purpose of Description, Exploration or Explanation.

- Survey research is defined as "the collection of information from a sample of individuals through their responses to questions." (Check and Schutt, 2012).
- Survey research is used "to answer questions that have been raised, to solve problems that have been posed or observed, to assess needs and set goals, to determine whether or not specific objectives have been met, to establish baselines against which future comparisons can be made, to analyze trends across time, and generally, to describe what exists, in what amount, and in what context." (Isaac and Michael, 1997).
- Pinsonneault and Kraemer (1993) defined survey as a "means for gathering information about the characteristics, actions, or opinions of a large group of people."

CORNERSTONES OF SURVEY RESEARCH (FIG. 15.1)

Specification: Specification of the research question and the drafting of survey questions are conceptual and very much concerned with the construct validity of the measurement.

Coverage error: When some members of the population have a zero probability of being selected in the survey sample.

Sampling error: Only a subset of people in the population is actually surveyed.

Nonresponse error: When some of the sampled units do not respond and when these units differ from those who do and in a way relevant to the study.

Measurement error: When a respondent's answer to a question is inaccurate, away from the "true" value.

CHARACTERISTICS OF GOOD SURVEY RESEARCH

Kraemer (1991) identified three distinguishing characteristics of survey research. First, survey research is mainly used to quantitatively describe specific aspects of population of interest by the researcher and checking the relationships among variables. Second, the survey researches data are collected from people are subjective. Finally, survey research findings from a selected portion of the population can later be generalized back to the population. In survey research,

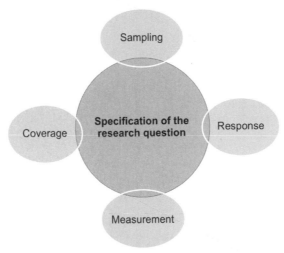

Figure 15.1: Cornerstones of survey research.

independent and dependent variables are used to define the scope of study, but cannot be explicitly controlled by the researcher. Before conducting the survey, the researcher must identify the expected relationships among these variables. The survey is then constructed to test this model against observations of the phenomena.

Survey research is popular because of its versatility, efficiency, and generalizability. Surveys are efficient as many variables can be measured and data can be collected from many people in less time or cost. Survey researches are predominantly cross-sectional in nature, at a specific point of time. However, longitudinal prospective or retrospective surveys are also not uncommon. Longitudinal retrospective surveys use data from already documented records. Readers must be familiar with survey during polls in predicting the expected result of a poll and is a practical example to keep in mind the survey research and the analysis conducted around a political election. Survey research in medical research is similar to it but the intended applications may vary. Predominantly survey research finds their use in policy decision. The basic characteristics of a good survey research design are shown in Figure 15.2.

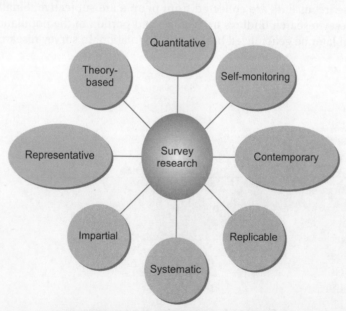

Figure 15.2: Characteristics of good survey research.

SURVEY TOOL

"A good question is one that produces answers that are reliable and valid measures of something we want to describe." (Fowler, 1995).

In survey to ensure that possibly relevant questions are asked is to use questions suggested by prior research, theory, experience, or experts. Moreover, the survey researchers also use a technique for improving questions called the **cognitive interview** (Dillman, 2007). By listening to and observing the focus group discussions, researchers can validate their assumptions of what people are going to be reporting. Conducting a pilot study is the final stage of questionnaire preparation. Complete the questionnaire and then revise it as it demands. The different types of survey tool is shown in Box 15.1.

Box 15.1: Survey tool

Questionnaire: A survey instrument containing the questions in a self-administered survey.
Interview schedule: A survey instrument containing the questions asked by the interviewer in an in-person or phone survey.
Closed-Ended and Open-Ended Questions.

The survey questionnaire may include the following type of questions: Dichotomous Question, Multiple Choice Question, Rank Order Scaling, Semantic Differential Scale, Likert Scale, Constant Sum Question, Open-Ended Question, Demographic Questions.

ADVANTAGES OF SURVEY

Surveys are capable of obtaining information from large samples of the population and capable of gathering demographic data that describe the composition of the sample. Surveys require minimal investment to develop and administer, and are relatively easy for making generalizations. Surveys can also be useful in collecting information about attitudes that are otherwise difficult to measure using observational techniques. But it is important to understand that surveys can only provide estimates for the true population, not exact measurements. The main advantages of survey research for a researcher are given below:

- Quickness
- Inexpensiveness
- Flexibility
- Efficiency

- Accuracy
- Helpful in the decision-making process.

SURVEY DESIGNS

1. Mail survey: A **mailed survey** is conducted by mailing a question-naire to respondents, who then administer the survey themselves. The central concern in a mailed survey is maximizing the response rate. Even an attractive questionnaire full of clear questions requires additional efforts to maximize the response rate. A response rate of 70% or higher is desirable and acceptable for data analysis.

2. Phone survey: It is done using random digit dialling, allows fast turnaround and efficient sampling. Multiple callbacks are often required, and the rate of nonresponse to phone interviews is rising.

3. In person survey: They allow longer and more complex interview schedules, monitoring of the conditions when the questions are answered, probing for respondents' understanding of the questions, and high response rates. However, the interviewer must balance the need to establish rapport with the respondent with the importance of maintaining control over the delivery of the interview questions.

4. Web survey (electronic survey): It can be fast and efficient for populations with high rates of computer use.

5. Mixed mode surveys: Mixed-mode surveys allow the strengths of one survey design to compensate for the weaknesses of another.

CLASSIFICATION OF SURVEY RESEARCH METHODS

Surveys can be classified according to the mode of communication, type of questions asked to the respondents or the time frame taken to collect the data.

Table 15.1: Classification of survey research methods

According to the mode of communication	Personal interviews, telephone interviews, mail surveys, internet surveys
According to the type of questions	Structured and disguised questions Closed-ended and open-ended questions
According to the time frame	Cross-sectional and longitudinal survey

SURVEY PROCESS

The survey research process is not that easy to meet the desired goals or perfection until and unless it is planned and executed properly, otherwise it may be a flop show at the end. It is a much more complex procedure than simply asking questions and compiling answers to produce statistics. There are numerous steps to be carried out following precise methods and procedures. These steps include formulating the survey objectives, determining the sample design, designing the questionnaire, performing data collection, processing and tabulating data and disseminating results. According to Groves, et al survey methodology 2004, the survey process includes the following steps:

1. Define the research objectives of the survey
2. Choose sampling frame and method of data collection
3. Select the sample
4. Construct the tool or questionnaire
5. Pre-test the questionnaire
6. Measurement, coding and editing of data
7. Analysis of data
8. Data dissemination
9. Documentation

DETERMINATION OF SAMPLE SIZE IN SURVEY

Determination of sample size in survey research depends on the following factors:

1. Desired degree of precision
   a. Significance level is the amount of Type I error that the researcher will allow in the study-5% level is normally preferred
   b. Confidence interval-95% confident statistic for the population falls within the specified range of the sample statistic.
2. Statistical power required-Statistical power is the probability that the researcher rejects the null hypothesis given that the alternate hypothesis is true (minimum of 80% power is necessary).
3. Ability of the researcher to gain access to the study subjects.

4. Degree to which the population can be stratified
5. Selection of the relevant units of analysis

   The sample size determination attempts to control for sampling errors and for nonresponse that occurs randomly. It does not attempt to control for other non-sampling errors.

Sample Size Formula

Sample size formula is described in Table 15.2.

Precision of an Estimated Proportion; Any Sample Design (When the Response Rate is <100%)

A physiotherapist wants to obtain an estimate of the overall satisfaction of the patients who attended OPD in the year 2016. It would not be possible to contact all the 1,500 patients because of time restrictions, the therapist has decided to interview a simple random sample by telephone.

Assumptions for this example include:

- The therapist will be satisfied if the true population proportion is within ±0.10 of the estimated population proportion based on the sample results, i.e. the required margin of error, e, is 0.10;
- The therapist wishes to have a level of confidence of 95% in the survey estimates (this means there would only be a 1 in 20 chance of getting a sample that produces an estimate outside the range $\hat{P} \pm .10$, therefore, $z = 1.96$.);
- Simple random sampling(SRS) will be used;
- A response rate of approximately 75% is expected, so $r = .75$;
- There is no advance estimate of $\hat{P}$, the level of patient satisfaction, consequently, $\hat{P} = .5$ is assumed.

The required sample size is calculated as follows:

1. Calculate the initial sample size, n_1:

$$n_1 = \frac{z^2 \hat{P}(1 - \hat{p})}{e^2}$$

$$n_1 = \frac{(1.96)^2(.50)(.50)}{(.10)^2} = 96$$

2. Adjust the sample size to account for the size of the population:

$$n_2 = n_1 \frac{N}{N + n_1}$$

$$n_2 = 96 \frac{1500}{1500 + 96} = 90$$

Table 15.2: Sample size formula

Precision of an estimated average	Precision of an estimated proportion	Precision of an estimated proportion
Simple Random Sample (100% Response)	Simple Random Sample (100% Response)	Any Sample Design (When the Response Rate is <100%)
$$n = \dfrac{z^2 \hat{S}^2}{e^2 + \dfrac{z^2 \hat{S}^2}{N}}$$	$$n = \dfrac{z^2 \hat{P}(1 - \hat{P})}{e^2 + \dfrac{z^2 \hat{P}(1 - \hat{P})}{N}}$$	initial sample size $$n_1 = \dfrac{z^2 \hat{P}(1 - \hat{P})}{e^2}$$ **adjusted for the size of the population** $$n_2 = n_1 \dfrac{N}{N + n_1}$$ **adjusted for the design effect** $$n_3 = \text{deff} \times n_2$$ *deff* is the design effect and usually: *deff* = 1 for simple random sampling designs; *deff* < 1 for stratified sampling designs; *deff* > 1 for cluster or multi-stage sample designs **adjusted for the response rate** $$n = \dfrac{n_3}{r}$$ *r* is the expected response rate.
a desired margin of error, *e*; • a value corresponding to a desired level of confidence, *z* • the size of the population, *N*; • an estimate of the population variability, $\hat{S}_2$.	If, prior to the survey, a good estimate of the proportion, $\hat{P}$, is available, then it should be used in the above equation. Otherwise, if nothing is known about the population, $\hat{P}$ = .5 may be used, which yields the maximum sample size given the other assumptions	

3. Adjust the sample size for the effect of the sample design:
$$n_3 = deff \times n_2$$
$$n_3 = 1 \times 90 = 90$$
For this example, $deff = 1$ since it is assumed that an SRS will be used.

4. Adjust for response to determine the final sample size, n:
$$n = \frac{n_3}{r}$$
$$n = 90/.75 = 120$$

[**Note:** if a response rate of at least 75% is not achieved when the survey is conducted, the final sample size will be smaller than planned, and therefore, the survey estimates may be less precise than the planning requirement. If a higher response rate is realized, the resulting sample will be larger than anticipated, and survey estimates may be more precise.]

ERRORS IN SURVEY RESEARCH

1. Errors of observation
2. Errors of non-observation

1. Errors of observation

Errors of observation stem from the way questions are written, the characteristics of the respondents who answer the questions, the way questions are presented in questionnaires, and the interviewers used to ask the questions. Measurement errors associated with Surveys may be due to the following issues:

• *Lengthy wording* (long and complicated), *Length of question* (unnecessarily long), *Lack of specificity*, *Lack of frame of reference* and *Vague language*.
• *Double negatives:* The Question uses two or more negative phrases.
• *Double barrelled:* There *is* two or more questions.
• Phrasing uses professional or academic discipline-specific terminologies.
• *Leading questions* (meant to bias the response).
• *Cultural differences in meaning:* Phrases or words have different meanings to different population subgroups.
• *Memory recall* (Problems remembering events or details about events).
• *Telescoping* Remembering events as happening more recently than when they really occurred.
• *Agreement bias* (Tendency for respondents to "agree".)

- *Social desirability* (Tendency of providing the desirable response).
- *Floaters (Respondents* choose a substantive answer).
- *Fence-sitters* (being neutral so as not to give the wrong answer).
- *Sensitive questions* (too personal).
- *Open-ended questions:* Response categories are not provided, left to respondent to provide.
- *Closed-ended questions:* Possible response categories are provided.
- *Agree-disagree:* Tendency to agree when only two choices are offered.
- *Order of the question:* The context or order of questions can affect subsequent responses as respondents try to remain consistent.
- *Response set:* Giving the same response to a series of questions.
- *Filter questions:* Questions used to determine if other questions are relevant.

2. **Errors of non-observation**
   - Due to a poor sampling frame
   - Sampling error
   - Nonresponse to specific question.

There are other two types of survey errors – sampling error and non-sampling errors.

Sampling errors	Non-sampling errors
Sampling error arises from estimating a population characteristic by measuring only a portion of the population rather than the entire population	Non-sampling errors can be defined as errors arising during the course of virtually all survey activities, apart from sampling
Frame error Chance error Response error	Coverage error Measurement error Nonresponse error Processing error

In addition to the errors in survey research, researchers also need to be aware of common biases in survey research. As responders are the key to a survey research, the bias that surrounds this type of research is mostly responder related bias. Some common responder bias are volunteer bias, social desirability, deviation, faking good, faking bad, positive and negative skew, end aversion or central tendency bias.

SURVEY RESEARCH EXAMPLES IN PHYSIOTHERAPY

Some examples of research titles on survey research is mentioned below:

1. Satisfaction with outpatient physiotherapy—survey of patients with MSK conditions.
2. Effect of a new electrotherapy machine on reducing swelling in legs—physiotherapy practitioner's survey.
3. Professional satisfaction among middle aged Physiotherapist clinicians in hospitals – a cross-sectional survey.

1. Hiscock A, et al. Frequency and circumstances of falls in people with inclusion body myositis: a questionnaire survey to explore falls management and physiotherapy provision. Physiotherapy, 2014;100(1):61-65.
2. V Panhale P, Bellare B, Jiandani M. Evidence-based practice in Physiotherapy curricula: A survey of Indian Health Science Universities. Journal of advances in medical education and professionalism. 2017;5(3):101-7.
3. Sullivan M, et al. Understanding North American yoga therapists' attitudes, skills and use of evidence-based practice: A cross-national survey. Complement Ther Med, 2017;32:11-18.
4. Green M, Norman KE. Knowledge and Use of, and Attitudes toward, Non-Steroidal Anti-Inflammatory Drugs (NSAIDs) in Practice: A Survey of Ontario Physiotherapists. Physiother Can, 2016;68(3):230-41.

FURTHER READING

1. Check J, Schutt RK. Survey research. In: Check J, Schutt RK (Eds). Research methods in education. Thousand Oaks, CA: Sage Publications; 2012. pp. 159–85.
2. Dillman DA, Smyth JD, Christian LM. Internet, phone, mail, and mixed-mode surveys: The tailored design method. Hoboken, NJ: John Wiley and Sons, Inc; 2014.
3. Ponto J. Understanding and evaluating survey research. Journal of the Advanced Practitioner in Oncology. 2015;6(2):168-71.

PART 2

Statistics in Research

+ Descriptive and Inferential Statistics in Research
+ Hypothesis Testing
+ Nonparametric and Parametric Tests
+ Correlation, Regression and Multivariate Analysis
+ Interpretation of Statistics.

16 Descriptive and Inferential Statistics in Research

STATISTICS

The word 'Statistics' is derived from the Latin word *Status*, means a political state. Statistics is concerned with scientific methods for collecting, organizing, summarizing, presenting and analyzing data as well as deriving valid conclusions and making reasonable decisions on the basis of this analysis. The fundamental reason behind statistics in scientific research is that "it enables scientist to make a numerical evaluation of the uncertainty in his conclusion", thus, paving way for an abstract towards real meaning.

DEFINITIONS

The following few definitions describe statistics from different view points:

- Statistics are numerical statement of facts in any department of enquiry placed in relation to each other. **— A.L. Bowley**
- Statistics may be defined as the science of collection, presentation analysis and interpretation of numerical data from the logical analysis. **— Croxton and Cowden**
- Statistics may be defined as the aggregate of facts affected to a marked extent by multiplicity of causes, numerically expressed, enumerated or estimated according to a reasonable standard of accuracy, collected in a systematic manner, for a predetermined purpose and placed in relation to each other. **— Horace Secrist**

FUNCTIONS OF STATISTICS

From the values or codes deduced from statistics, it is said that in short, there are some specific functions of statistics:

- Condensation: Classification and tabulation of data.
- Comparison: Grand totals, measures of central tendency, measures of dispersion, graphs and diagrams, coefficient of correlation are useful for comparison.
- Forecasting: To predict (time series and regression analysis plays an important role in forecasting).
- Estimation: Estimate the unknown value of the population parameter based on the sample observations.
- Tests of hypothesis: Statistical methods/tests are extremely useful in hypothesis testing.

BASIC ARITHMETIC

Numerical deduction of values in statistics need a basic knowledge of following simple operations in arithmetic and its understanding is necessary for the researcher; otherwise the results may be misleading or wrongly perceived.

Decimals: Derived from addition, subtraction, multiplication, division
Fractions
Negative numbers: Derived from addition, subtraction, multiplication, division
Exponents
Proportions and percentages
Rounding numbers
Removing parentheses

BASIC CONCEPTS

A parameter is a characteristic of a population and a statistic is a characteristic of a sample. A researcher can describe samples and populations by using measures such as the mean, median, mode and standard deviation.

Population: The whole set of a "universe". It could be finite population or infinite population.

Sample: A sub-set of a population.

Parameter: An unknown "fixed" value of population characteristic.

Statistic: A known/calculable value of sample characteristic representing that of the population.

The Symbols used for Parameters and Statistics

Characteristic	Parameter	Statistic
Mean	μ	$\bar{x}$
Standard deviation	σ	s
Variance	σ2	S^2
Proportion	ρ	p
Pearson correlation coefficient	R	γ
Number of cases	n	N

TYPES OF DATA

The data that are generated in statistics can be grouped into the following for ease of calculation and inference description.

Qualitative Data

Nominal data (binary), e.g. Male/female, present/not present, affected/unaffected, etc.
Nominal data (multi-categorical), e.g. Income groups, social class, etc.
Ranked data (categorical), e.g. Mild, moderate, severe spasticity.
Ranked data (continuous), e.g. Visual analogue scale scores.

Quantitative Data

Numerical data (discrete), e.g. Number of joints, number of falls, etc.
Numerical data (continuous), e.g. Age, height, weight, etc.

METHODS OF PRESENTATION OF DATA

The collected data could be presented by the following methods in research:
1. Tabulation: Simple tables, frequency distribution tables.
2. Charts and diagrams: Pie diagram, simple and multiple bar charts, line graphs, scatter diagram, histogram, and frequency polygon, cumulative frequency diagram (Ogive), map diagram and pictogram.

DESCRIPTIVE STATISTICS

It is a summary statistics which quantitatively describes the features of the collected data. It is capable of only describing the sample it has got nothing to do with population as is in inferential statistics. The commonly used descriptive to describe a data set are:

1. Measures of central tendency (Mean, median and mode)
2. Measures of variability (Variance and standard deviation)
3. Measures of dispersion (Kurtosis and skewness)
4. Measures for size of the distribution (Maximum, minimum, range and sum)
5. Measures of stability (Standard error).

Common Descriptive Statistics

Common descriptive statistics are described in Table 16.1.

Table 16.1: Common descriptive statistics

Count (frequencies)	Total number of items
Percentage	Per hundred
Central tendency	In the study of a population it is not possible to grasp any idea about the characteristic when we look at all the observations. A representative number can be a central value for all these observations.
Mean	Mean of a variable is defined as the sum of the observations divided by the number of observations.
Mode	The mode refers to that value in a distribution, which occur most frequently.
Median	The median is that value which divides the group into two equal parts, one part comprising all values greater, and the other, all values less than median.
Range	A measure of dispersion and is defined as the difference between the largest and smallest values of the variable.
Inter quartile range	It is a statistical measure describing the extent of middle 50% of ranked data.
Standard deviation/ Root-Mean Square deviation	It is defined as the positive square-root of the arithmetic mean of the Square of the deviations of the given observation from their arithmetic mean (sigma). $$\sigma = \sqrt{\left(\frac{\Sigma x^2}{n}\right)} \text{ or } \sqrt{\frac{\Sigma(X - \bar{X})^2}{n}}$$
Mean deviation/ Average deviation	Mean deviation is the arithmetic mean of the deviations of a series computed from any measure of central tendency. Average deviation is the average amount scatter of the items in a distribution from either the mean or the median, ignoring the signs of the deviations.
Coefficient of mean deviation	(Mean deviation/mean or Median or Mode × 100

Contd...

Contd...

Count (frequencies)	Total number of items
Variance	Variance is the expectation of the squared deviation of a random variable from its mean. The square root of variance forms the standard deviation.
Coefficient of variation	It is obtained by dividing the standard deviation by the mean and multiply it by 100.
Ranking	A position in the hierarchy (grading).
Skewness	Skewness is a measure of asymmetry and shows the manner in which the items are clustered around the average.
Kurtosis	Kurtosis is the measure of flat-toppedness of a curve. A bell shaped curve or the normal curve is Mesokurtic because it is kurtic in the center; but if the curve is relatively more peaked than the normal curve, it is called Leptokurtic whereas a curve is more flat than the normal curve, it is called Platykurtic.
Normal distribution	Gaussian distribution-observations with moderate values have high frequencies than extreme values, a bell shaped curve.
Standard error	When time and again samples are taken from the same population the mean slightly differs for such samples. If there is a sampling distribution of means of all the samples, the standard deviation of such distribution is known as standard error.

Descriptive Statistics for a Sample Data

Data: (n = 7): [5.00, 7.00, 9.00, 3.00, 6.00, 8.00, 6.00]

Mean = (5 + 7 + 9 + 3 + 6 + 8 + 6)/7 = 6.285

Median = 3, 5, 6, <u>6,</u> 7, 8, 9 = 6

Mode = 3, 5, <u>6, 6,</u> 7, 8, 9 = 6

Maximum = 9

Minimum = 3

Range = 6

Sum = 5 + 7 + 9 + 3 + 6 + 8 + 6 = 44

Kurtosis = .185

Skewness = –.370

Standard error = .746

Variance = 3.905

Standard deviation = 1.976

Example of Descriptive Statistics in a Research Study

Tables 16.2 to 16.4 are the examples of descriptive statistics of a researcher presented in a study. They are given as frequencies, mean, standard deviation, etc. The reader can easily understand the tables as they are descriptive in nature.

Table 16.2: Frequencies of a study data

Subject characteristics	Level	Percentage (%)
Education	Illiterate School Higher study	3.4 47.5 49.2
Occupation	Unemployed Employed Business	27.1 28.8 44.1
HTC use (Hemophilia treatment center)	Frequent Infrequent Rare	20.3 22.0 57.6
Factor level	<1 >1	86.4 13.6
Inhibitor	No Yes	81.4 18.6
Mode of treatment	Minimal transfusion Episodic transfusion E/H	3.4 94.9 1.7
Pain	No pain Mild pain Moderate pain Severe pain	8.5 27.1 62.7 1.7
Bleeding	No bleeding Mild bleeding Moderate bleeding	6.8 66.1 27.1
Total joint score	Mild Moderate Severe	16.9 44.1 39.0

Table 16.3: Mean and standard deviations of variables of a study data

Clinical outcome	Mean	Standard deviation
WHO BREF QOL score		
Physical health (0-100) Psychological (0-100) Social relationship (0-100) Environment (0-100)	63.23 66.15 69.42 73.15	9.30 12.34 23.55 13.62
FUNCTIONAL INDEPENDENCE (FISH) score		
Self-care (3-12) Transfer (2-8) Locomotion (3-12) Total functional independence (8-32)	11.74 5.55 8.69 25.98	.658 1.27 1.92 2.93

Contd...

Contd...

Clinical outcome	Mean	Standard deviation
GILBERT JOINT score		
Pain (0-3)	1.58	.674
Bleeding (0-3)	1.20	.550
Total joint score (0-12)	7.85	3.22

Table16.4: Descriptive statistics of variables of a study data

N = 266	Range	Minimum	Maximum	Mean		Std. Deviation	Variance	Skewness		Kurtosis	
	Statistic	Statistic	Statistic	Statistic	Std. Error	Statistic	Statistic	Statistic	Std. Error	Statistic	Std. Error
Height (meter)	.44	1.35	1.79	1.59	.005	.082	.007	-.124	.149	-.483	.298
Weight (kg)	64.0	56.0	120.0	81.51	.661	10.792	116.477	.132	.149	-.272	.298
BMI	26.78	25.16	51.94	32.02	.277	4.522	20.455	1.265	.149	2.501	.298

INFERENTIAL STATISTICS

Inferential statistics helps the researcher to predict and judge the population through the sample data. It also can reveal the researcher that the difference exists between groups is real or due to probability of chance. Hypothesis testing using various statistical tests like parametric, non-parametric and regression analyses are under the category of inferential statistics. But they are not hundred percent accurate in prediction so the testing procedures are aimed to reduce the margin of error and calculate the error which is known as statistical estimation.

1. Estimation
2. Tests of hypothesis
3. Non-parametric/parametric tests
4. Sequential/Time series analysis.

Common Inferential Statistics

Tables 16.5 and 16.6 explain the inferential statistics where a hypothesis was tested whether there is a difference between male and females on their weight using independent *t test*. It showed that there was 8.317 kg difference between them with a statistical significance of p value = .000.

Table 16.5: Common Inferential statistics

Null hypothesis	**It is a statement regarding the value(s) of unknown parameter(s). Typically will imply no association between explanatory and response variables in our applications (will always contain an equality)**
Alternate hypothesis	It is the proposed experimental hypothesis. A Statement contradictory to the null hypothesis (will always contain an inequality)
Type I error	**Type I error** is the probability of rejecting a null hypothesis that is actually true.
p-value	A *p* value is the probability of obtaining a sample outcome, given that the value stated in the null hypothesis is true.
Significance	A criterion of judgment upon which a decision is made regarding the value stated in a null hypothesis. The criterion is based on the probability of obtaining a statistic measured in a sample if the value stated in the null hypothesis were true (level of significance is typically set at 5% in research studies).

Contd...

Contd...

Type II error	**Type II error** is the probability of accepting a null hypothesis that is actually not true.
Power	The **power** in hypothesis testing is the probability of rejecting a false null hypothesis.
Sample size calculation	It is the size or number of subjects needed for a research study and which is calculated by using formulae according to the study design and many other factors.
Standard error of measurement	The standard error of measurement (SEm) is a measure of how much measured test scores are spread around a "true" score. It is the repeated measures of a person on the same instrument tend to be distributed around his or her "true" score.
Confidence interval	A Confidence Interval is a **range of values** within which the **true value** lies in.

LIST OF STATISTICAL PACKAGES

There are many statistical packages which are specialized computer programs for analysis in statistics. Statistical packages can be used for Data Analysis, Data Manipulation and Data Management. Different statistical packages have different strengths at the level of application. So the researchers should acquire knowledge through adequate training before using them in their study. Among many good statistical packages which are now available, the choice always depends on the packages which are normally supported by the particular organization. Researchers must be interested to use one of the dedicated statistical packages, rather than a spread sheet as they have a wider range of statistical methods, optimized algorithms and the manuals which often provide more help with the interpretation of the results than is available with a spread sheet. It is easy to paste material from a spread sheet into a statistical package, so if the researcher wants, the raw data can be kept in the spread sheet.

The researchers can access the following link to know about the strengths of various statistical packages: https://en.wikipedia.org/wiki/Comparison_of_statistical_packages. Very commonly used are mentioned in Table 16.7.

Table 16.6: Inferential statistics of a research study

Group Statistics

	Sex	N	Mean	Std. Deviation	Std. Error Mean
Weight	Male	147	85.236	9.2651	.7642
	Female	119	76.924	10.8105	.9910

Independent Samples Test

		Levene's Test for Equality of Variances		t-test for Equality of Means						
		F	Sig.	t	df	Sig. (2-tailed)	Mean Difference	Std. Error Difference	95% Confidence Interval of the Difference	
									Lower	Upper
Weight	Equal variances assumed	4.654	.032	6.750	264	.000	8.3117	1.2313	5.8872	10.7362
	Equal variances not assumed			6.642	233.364	.000	8.3117	1.2514	5.8462	10.7772

Table 16.7 describes the common statistical packages available through internet.

Table 16.7: Statistical packages

Source	Statistical packages
Open-source	Gretl, Matlab, PSPP – A free software alternative to IBM SPSS Statistics, R Commander, R studio, Statistical Lab
Public domain	CSPro, Epi Info
Freeware	MaxStat Lite, MINUIT
Proprietary	Analytica, Graph Pad InStat, MATLAB, Maple, Minitab, PASS, SPSS, Stata and SAS

LIMITATIONS OF STATISTICS

Statistics is not suitable to the study of qualitative phenomenon

- Statistics does not study individuals
- Statistical laws are not exact
- Statistics may be misused
- Statistical study should be supplemented by other evidences.

FURTHER READING

1. Ali Z, Bhaskar SB. Basic statistical tools in research and data analysis. Indian Journal of Anaesthesia. 2016;60(9),662–9. http://doi.org/10.4103/0019-5049.190623.
2. Binu, V, et al. Some basic aspects of statistical methods and sample size determination in health science research. AYU (An international quarterly journal of research in Ayurveda) 2014;35(2):119-123.
3. Bland M. An Introduction to Medical Statistics, 2nd ed. England: Oxford University Press; 1995.
4. Daniel WW. Biostatistics: A Foundation for Analysis in Health Sciences, 7th ed. Singapore, Asia: John Wiley and Sons Pte. Ltd.; 2004.
5. Larson MG. Descriptive statistics and graphical displays. Circulation 2006;114:76-81.

Hypothesis Testing

HYPOTHESIS TESTING OR SIGNIFICANCE TESTING

Researchers use inferential statistics to measure behavior or outcome in samples in order to learn more about the behavior or outcome in populations which are often too large and very difficult to access. In a study the researchers measure a sample mean to learn more about the mean in a population. The method in which the samples selected to learn more about characteristics in a given population is called hypothesis testing. **Hypothesis testing** is an important activity of empirical research.

Hypothesis testing or **significance testing:** It is a method for testing a statement or hypothesis about a parameter in a population, using the data measured through a sample.

FOUR STEPS TO HYPOTHESIS TESTING

Step 1	State the hypotheses
Step 2	Set the criteria for a decision
Step 3	Compute the test statistic
Step 4	Make a decision

STEP 1 HYPOTHESIS (NULL HYPOTHESIS VS. ALTERNATIVE HYPOTHESIS)

According to philosopher Karl Popper (1976) the first important step of scientific process is not observation, it is the generation of a hypothesis which can be tested by observations and experiments. Popper also claims that the main aim of the researcher is not the verification of hypothesis but the falsification of the initial hypothesis.

"It is logically impossible to verify the truth of a general law by repeated observations, but, at least in principle, it is possible to falsify such a law by a single observation. Repeated observations of white swans did not prove that all swans are white, but the observation of a single black swan sufficed to falsify that general statement".

Hypothesis

It is a claim or statement about a property of a population/a guess from the researcher. It is also otherwise called as the assumption the researcher on the particular property the researcher intends to study.

According to Hulley et al., 2001 a good hypothesis is based on a good research question. It should be simple, specific and stated in advance.

"Hypothesis is a formal statement that presents the expected relationship between an independent and dependent variable." (Creswell, 1994).

Good characteristics of a hypothesis:

Basically a good hypothesis should have the following features:

- Clearly written and concise
- Susceptible to observation
- Amenable to testing within a reasonable time
- State the relationship between the independent and dependent variables
- Capable of predicting on an outcome
- Should have empirical reference
- Falsifiable.

Basically the research hypotheses are of four types: Null, directional, non-directional and causal (Table 17.1).

Table 17.1: Types of hypothesis

Null hypothesis	There is no significant difference of groups compared in the study.
Non-directional hypothesis	There is a relationship between the variables compared, but do not specify the exact nature of this relationship.
Directional hypothesis	There is a relationship between the variables compared and suggests the outcome what is expected at the end of the study.
Causal hypothesis	This hypothesis states the effect of a particular factor or variable on another factor.

Null Hypothesis

It is a statement regarding the value of unknown parameter. Typically there is no association between explanatory and response variables of the study and will always contain an equality. It is the primary assumption on which the whole statistical calculation is based on. A research starts with an assumption that there is no association between the variables that we are interested in and try to prove that statistically. If the null hypothesis is false then our assumption that there is no association is also wrong hence be rejected. In other words alternative hypothesis is true (Table 17.2).

Alternative Hypothesis

It is the proposed experimental hypothesis. A Statement contradictory to the null hypothesis and will always contain an inequality. It means that there is an association between the variables of interest proved based on the statistical rejection of null hypothesis (Table 17.2).

One or Two Tailed Hypothesis (Fig. 17.1)

In hypothesis testing significance tests may be used to examine only one direction of the alternative hypothesis, **disregarding the opposite direction.** Meaning, when hypothesis is tested only in one direction that either one among the Null or Alternative is true. These are called 'one-tailed significance tests'. Alternatively, significance tests when it did not make any assumptions about the direction of difference (examining both directions) of the null and alternative. These are 'two-tailed significance tests'. One-tailed tests are less preferred than two-tailed tests and should only be used in situations where one of the directions of difference has been proved to be implausible.

Table 17.2: Difference between null hypothesis and alternative hypothesis

Null Hypothesis	Alternative Hypothesis
<ul><li>Statement about the value of a population parameter</li><li>Represented by H0</li><li>Always stated as an Equality</li></ul>	<ul><li>Statement about the value of a population parameter that must be true if the null hypothesis is false</li><li>Represented by H1</li><li>Stated in three forms<ul><li>– ></li><li>– <</li><li>– ≠</li></ul></li></ul>

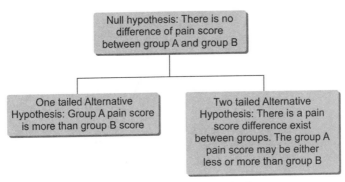

Figure 17.1: One or two tailed hypothesis.

STEP 2 LEVEL OF SIGNIFICANCE

Level of significance, or significance level, refers to a criterion of judgment upon which a decision is made regarding the value stated in a null hypothesis. The criterion is based on the probability of obtaining a statistic measured in a sample if the value stated in the null hypothesis were true whether our assumption at the start of the research is true.

The likelihood or level of significance is typically set at 5% in research studies. By 5% means, one in out of 20, there is a probability that the null hypothesis is rejected in the research that is undertaken. Also, it is to be said that rejecting null hypothesis on the basis of a probability of 1 in 20 is fairer than 1 in 2, i.e. 0.05 against 0.5.

When the probability of obtaining a sample mean is less than 5% if the null hypothesis were true, then we conclude that the sample we selected is too unlikely and so we reject the null hypothesis.

STEP 3 THE TEST STATISTIC

The **test statistic** is a mathematical formula that allows researchers to determine the likelihood of obtaining sample outcomes if the null hypothesis were true or in other words The value of the test statistic is used to make a decision regarding the null hypothesis.

Specifically, a test statistic tells us how far, or how many standard deviations, a sample mean (x) is from the population mean (μ). The larger the value of the test statistic, the further the distance, or number of standard deviations, a sample mean is from the population mean stated in the null hypothesis (Fig. 17.2). The closeness derived between

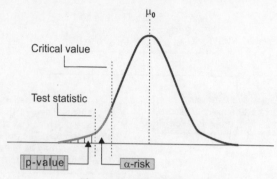

Figure 17.2: Test statistic.

sample mean from many random samples and population mean is purely by chance and the fact that both the means are close depends on two factors. One is the variability of sample means in general population and sample size. This is the inference that a research would provide about the variable of interest that we are interested in studying.

STEP 4 DECISION MAKING

1. Reject the null hypothesis. The sample mean is associated with a low probability of occurrence when the null hypothesis is true.
2. Retain the null hypothesis. The sample mean is associated with a high probability of occurrence when the null hypothesis is true.

   A *p* **value** is the probability of obtaining a sample outcome, given that the value stated in the null hypothesis is either true or false. The *p* value for obtaining a sample outcome is compared to the level of significance.

   Significance, or **statistical significance**, describes a decision made concerning a value stated in the null hypothesis. When the null hypothesis is rejected, we reach significance. When the null hypothesis is retained, we fail to reach significance.

   Researchers make decisions regarding the null hypothesis. The decision can be to retain the null (p > .05) or reject the null (p < .05).

TYPES OF ERROR

Table 17.3 describes the four situations when a null hypothesis can be accepted are rejected. Errors in statistics are related to retaining or rejecting null hypothesis when vice versa is true. However situations arises listing as **errors** when incorrect decisions are possible.

1. The researcher's decision to retain the null hypothesis could be correct.
2. The researcher's decision to retain the null hypothesis could be incorrect.
3. The researcher's decision to reject the null hypothesis could be correct.
4. The researcher's decision to reject the null hypothesis could be incorrect.

Type I error is the probability of rejecting a null hypothesis that is actually true. Researchers directly control for the probability of committing this type of error.

An **alpha (α) level** is the level of significance or criterion for a hypothesis test. It is the largest probability of committing a Type I error that we will allow and still decide to reject the null hypothesis. Retain a true null hypothesis.

Type II error is the probability of accepting a null hypothesis that is actually not true.

The **power** in hypothesis testing is the probability of rejecting a false null hypothesis. Specifically, it is the probability that a randomly selected sample will show that the null hypothesis is false when the null hypothesis is indeed false.

The correct decision is to reject a false null hypothesis.

Table 17.3: Types of error

	Null hypothesis ↓	
Decision of researcher ↓	True	false
Accept	Correct decision	Type II error (beta)
Reject	Type I error (alpha)	Correct decision

HYPOTHESIS TESTING EXAMPLE

Goal: The researcher should make statement regarding unknown population parameter values based on sample data.

Elements of a hypothesis test: Null hypothesis, Alternative hypothesis, Test statistic rejection region.

Example: Efficacy test for new joint mobilization technique.

Null hypothesis (H_0): New joint mobilization technique is no better than standard conventional technique (there is no mean difference of the outcome measured to find the efficacy of both treatments).

Alternative hypothesis (H_A): New joint mobilization technique is better than standard conventional technique(there is a real mean difference of the outcome measured to find the efficacy of both treatments).

Sampling Distribution of difference in means: In large samples, the difference in two sample means is approximately normally distributed:

Type I error (Chance of ineffective new treatment is deemed better) probability is 5%; P = 0.05.

Type II error (Failing to conclude that the new effective treatment is deemed to be no better) probability is 20%; P ≤ .20

Test statistic: Through the difference between the sample means, standard deviation and sample size a test statistic 't'/'Z' calculated by using formula.

Decision making: Reject the null hypothesis if the observed Z value from formula greater than the table z value for alpha level .05

P-value: Measure of the strength of evidence the sample data provides against the null hypothesis. For the calculated Z value check the probability value.

Example:

- $H_0: \mu_1 - \mu_2 = 0$
- $H_A: \mu_1 - \mu_2 > 0$

- $T.S.: z_{obs} = \dfrac{10.1 - 7.7}{\sqrt{\dfrac{(3.6)^2}{33} + \dfrac{(3.4)^2}{35}}} = \dfrac{2.4}{0.85} = 2.82$

- $R.R.: z_{obs} \geq z_\alpha = z_{.05} = 1.645$
- $P - val: P(Z \geq 2.82) = .0024$

FURTHER READING

1. Banerjee A, Chitnis UB, Jadhav SL, Bhawalkar JS, Chaudhury S. Hypothesis testing, type I and type II errors. Industrial Psychiatry Journal, 2009;18(2), 127–31. http://doi.org/10.4103/0972-6748.62274.
2. Bland M. An introduction to medical statistics. Oxford: Oxford University Press, 1987.
3. Daniel WW. Hypothesis testing. In: Biostatistics. 7th ed. New York: John Wiley and Sons, Inc; 2002. pp. 204–94.

4. Davis RB, Mukamal KJ. Hypothesis Testing. Means 2006;114(10): 1078-82.
5. Guyatt G, Jaenschke R, Heddle N, Cook D, Shannon H, Walter S. Basic statistics for clinicians. Hypothesis testing. Can Med Assoc J 1995;152:27–32.
6. Sedgwick P. Understanding statistical hypothesis testing. BMJ: British Medical Journal, 2014; 348.

Non-parametric and Parametric Tests

STATISTICAL TESTS

Parametric and nonparametric are two broad classifications of statistical procedures which are used to analyze a data based on some assumptions. Compared to nonparametric tests the parametric analyses need to strictly follow some assumptions such as the shape or parameters of the sample distribution. The researchers must know how to evaluate the validity of those assumptions before making the decision of which test to be used and is always very difficult to make a decision between these two. In general, the nonparametric procedures have less power for the same sample size than the corresponding parametric procedure if the data is normally distributed. Moreover the interpretation of nonparametric procedures can also be more difficult than the parametric procedures. For small sample sizes (n < 30) nonparametric tests are often a good option.

The statistical analyses may for the following two purposes:

1. **Tests of significance:** It is used to address the question: what is the probability of relationship between two variables and is it really just a chance occurrence?
2. **Measures of association:** If it does, how strong is the relationship?

NONPARAMETRIC TESTS

Nonparametric tests are a class of statistical procedures that do not rely on assumptions about the shape or form of the probability distribution (normality) from which the data were drawn. They are specifically used when there is a skewed data. Because it is not always possible to have normality in a data as it is based on the sample size. With smaller sample size there is high probability of being a skewed data. There are advantages and disadvantages with nonparametric tests.

Advantages of Nonparametric Tests

- Used with all type of scales
- Easier to compute the statistics
- Make fewer assumptions
- Need not involve population parameters
- Results may be as exact as parametric procedures
- Used when sample sizes are small.

Disadvantages of Nonparametric Tests

- May waste information (Parametric model more efficient if data permit)
- Difficult to compute by hand for large samples
- Tables not widely available.

Assumptions

Nominal or ordinal data
Cannot be used to analyze differences in scores or their means
Expected frequencies should not be less than 5
No subjects can be count more than once.

TESTS OF SIGNIFICANCE—SELECTED NONPARAMETRIC TESTS

- *Chi-Square test:* For frequency data.
- *Fisher's exact test:* For N × N design and very small sample size Fisher's exact test should be applied.
- *McNemar test:* McNemar test can be used with two dichotomous measures on the same subjects (repeated measurements). It is used to measure change.
- *Mann-Whitney test:* Ordinal data independent groups.
- *Wilcoxon signed rank test:* Ordinal data dependent (paired samples) groups.
- *Kruskal-Wallis test:* Ordinal data independent groups (more than 2 groups).
- *Friedman test:* Ordinal data repeated measures.

Measures of Association
- Spearman correlation coefficient—for correlation of nonparametric data.

The following lists the nonparametric tests in situations when and where it should be used in the order of nominal and ordinal data.

The Chi-square Test (Table 18.1)
Conditions
- Any number of groups.
- Categorical data.
- Categorical data from different samples are compared (independence or relatedness).
- Categorical data from a single sample can be compared with a theoretical value (goodness of fit).
- No data point should be zero.

Null Hypothesis
No real differences exist between categorical data obtained from different samples, these samples belong to the same population.

Alternative Hypothesis
Real differences exist between categorical data obtained from compared samples.

Table 18.1: The chi-square test

	Group A (n=20)			Group B (n=20)		Group C (n=20)	
Is there a presence of fixed flexion deformity after elbow surgery?	Yes 12	No 8	Or / Vs	Yes 11	No 9	Yes 7	No 13

The Wilcoxon Rank Sum Test (Table 18.2)
Conditions
- One-sample data
- Skewed data
- Sample median is compared with a theoretical or hypothetical mean.

Null Hypothesis
Sample median derived belongs to the same population from which hypothetical mean was derived.

Alternative Hypothesis

Sample median is different from hypothetical mean that the Sample cannot be said to belong to the same population from which hypothetical mean was derived.

Table 18.2: The Wilcoxon rank sum test

Group (n=10)	Vs	Hypothetical mean (assumption by the researcher)
Median of perceived exertion of dyspnea score, e.g. 7/11		6/11

The Mann–Whitney U Test (Table 18.3)

Conditions

- Two independent samples
- Skewed/discrete data
- Unpaired data
- Sample a median (group A) is compared with Sample b (group B) median.

Null Hypothesis

Sample a median is not that different from Sample b median and both samples belong to the same population.

Alternative Hypothesis

Sample a median is too different from Sample b median for both samples to belong to the same population.

Table18.3: The Mann–Whitney U test

Group A (n=10)	Vs	Group B (n=10)
Median, e.g. pain score 6.5/10		Median, e.g. pain score 6/10

The Wilcoxon Matched-pairs Signed Rank Test (Table 18.4)

Conditions

- Two dependent samples
- Skewed/discrete data—paired data
- Sample median is compared before and after treatment.

Null Hypothesis

After treatment median is not different from before treatment median.

Alternative Hypothesis

After treatment median is different from before treatment median.

Table 18.4: The Wilcoxon matched-pairs signed rank test

Group A (n=10) Before treatment	Vs	Group A (n=10) After treatment
Median, e.g. pain score 6.5/10		Median, e.g. pain score 4.5/10

The Kruskal-Wallis Test (Table 18.5)

Conditions
- Three or more samples
- Skewed/discrete data
- Unpaired data
- Sample medians are compared from groups a, b, c,....

Null Hypothesis
No difference exists between the sample medians of all compared groups and they belong to the same population.

Alternative Hypothesis
A difference exists between the sample medians of all compared groups and too different samples also have come from the same population.

Table 18.5: The Kruskal-Wallis test

Group A (n=10)	Group B (n=10)	Group C (n=10)
Median, e.g. pain score 6.5/10	Median, e.g. pain score 5.5/10	Median, e.g. pain score 6/10

The Friedman Test (Table 18.6)

Conditions
- Three or more dependent samples
- Skewed/discrete data—paired data
- Sample median is compared for multiple level of measurements of the same sample.

Null Hypothesis
After treatment median is no different from before treatment median.

Alternative Hypothesis
After treatment median is different from before treatment median.

Table 18.6: The Friedman test

Group A (n=10) Before treatment	Group A (n=10) After 4 weeks treatment	Group A (n=10) After 8 weeks treatment
Median, e.g. pain score 6.5/10	Median, e.g. pain score 4.5/10	Median, e.g. pain score 3.5/10

PARAMETRIC TESTS

The parametric statistical procedures or tests mostly rely on few assumptions about the shape of the distribution (a normal distribution) in the underlying population and about the form or parameters (means and standard deviations) of the assumed distribution.

The following lists the advantages and disadvantages of parametric tests.

Advantages of Parametric Tests

- Powerful test to detect real difference
- Gives more information regarding the population as confidence intervals.

Disadvantages of Parametric Tests

- Not valid on very small data sets
- Useful only for interval or ratio scale data
- Size of sample is very big.

Assumptions

- Interval or ratio data
- Adequate sample size
- No subjects can belong to more than one group
- Equality of group variances (Homogeneity).

TESTS OF SIGNIFICANCE—SELECTED PARAMETRIC TESTS

- One group t-test: Comparison of sample mean with a population mean.
- Independent groups t-test: Comparison of means from two unrelated groups.
- Dependent or paired t-test: Comparison of means from two related samples.
- K unrelated group, one-way ANOVA test, two way ANOVA test: Comparison of means from K unrelated groups (more than 2 groups).
- Repeated measures ANOVA: Interval or ratio data repeated measures (Comparison of means from K related groups).

Measures of Association

- Pearson correlation coefficient: For correlation of parametric data.

The following lists the parametric tests in situations when and where it should be used to analyze the data.

The One-sample Test (Table 18.7)

Conditions
- One-sample data
- Normal data
- Sample mean is compared with a theoretical or hypothetical population mean.

Null Hypothesis

Sample from which mean was derived belongs to the same population from which population mean was derived.

Alternative Hypothesis

Sample mean is different from population mean that the sample cannot be said to belong to the same population from which population mean was derived.

Table18.7: The one-sample test

Group (n=100)	Vs	Hypothetical mean (assumption by the researcher)
Mean of quality of life score, e.g. 70		60 (cut off)

The t-test (Table 18.8)

Conditions
- Two independent samples
- Normal data
- Unpaired data.
- Sample mean of group A is compared with sample mean of group B.

Null Hypothesis

There is no difference between the group means and samples to belong to the same population.

Alternative Hypothesis

There is a real difference between the group means and samples to belong to the same population.

Table18.8: The *t*-test

Group A (n=60)	Vs	Group B (n=60)
Mean, e.g. pain score 6.5/10		Mean, e.g. pain score 6/10

The Paired t-test (Table 18.9)

Conditions
- Two samples
- Normal data

- Paired data
- The sample mean is compared before and after treatment.

Null Hypothesis
The after treatment mean is no different from before treatment mean.

Alternative Hypothesis
The after treatment mean is different from before treatment mean.

Table18.9: The paired *t*-test

Group A (n=60) Before treatment	Vs	Group A (n=60) After treatment
Mean, e.g. pain score 6.5/10		Mean, e.g. pain score 4.5/10

The Analysis of Variance (ANOVA) Test (Table 18.10)
Conditions
- Three or more samples
- Normal data
- Unpaired data
- Sample means are compared from groups a, b, c,...,

Null Hypothesis
No difference exists between the compared groups, all belong to the same population.

Alternative Hypothesis
A real difference exists between the compared groups and the groups do not come from the same population.

Table 18.10: The analysis of variance (ANOVA) test

Group A (n=30)	Group B (n=30)	Group C (n=30)
Mean, e.g. pain score 6.5/10	Mean, e.g. pain score 5.5/10	Mean, e.g. pain score 6/10

PARAMETRIC *VS* NONPARAMETRIC TESTS (TABLE 18.11)

Table 18.11: Parametric *vs* nonparametric tests

Parametric test procedures	Nonparametric test procedures
1. Involve population parameters (Mean)	1. Do not involve population parameters Example: Probability distributions, independence
2. Have stringent assumptions (Normality)	2. Data measured on any scale (Ratio or interval, ordinal or nominal)
3. Examples: Z Test, *t* test, F test	3. Example: Wilcoxon rank sum test

PARAMETRIC TESTS AND ANALOGOUS NONPARAMETRIC PROCEDURES (TABLE 18.12)

Table 18.12: Parametric tests and analogous nonparametric procedures

Type of analysis	Example	Parametric tests	Nonparametric tests
Compare means between two independent groups	Is the mean quality of life score of incontinence patients (at baseline) for patients assigned to placebo different from the mean for patients assigned to the treatment (Interferential therapy) group?	Two-sample t-test	Wilcoxon rank-sum test
Compare two quantitative repeated measurements taken from the same sample	Was there a significant change in Quality of life score of incontinence patients between baseline and the Four-month follow-up measurement in the treatment group?	Paired t-test	Wilcoxon signed-rank test
Compare means between three or more independent groups	If the study have three groups (e.g. placebo, Interferential therapy, Kegal's exercises), to know the mean difference among the three groups?	Analysis of variance (ANOVA)	Kruskal-Wallis test
Association between two quantitative variables	Is Quality of life score associated with the patient's age?	Pearson coefficient of correlation	Spearman's rank correlation

FURTHER READING

1. Altman D. Practical statistics for medical research. London: Chapman and Hall, 1995;210–2
2. Bland M. An introduction to medical statistics. Oxford: Oxford University Press, 1987.
3. Greenhalgh T. Statistics for the non-statistician. I. Different types of data need different statistical tests. BMJ 1997;315:000–0.

19   Correlation, Regression and Multivariate Analysis

CORRELATION

Correlation refers to the relationship of two variables or more. It measures and analyses the degree or extent to which the two variables vary with reference to each other. Correlation does not indicate cause and effect relationship. Correlation finds it best use when both compared variables have simply been measured and their values have not been controlled or pre-set in any way. For example, if variables such as Range of motion and functional outcome were measured in a randomly selected sample, correlation can be used to test for a possible linear association that may exist between them. The magnitude and direction of any identified linear associations are expressed as a correlation co-efficient. A positive correlation means that Y increases linearly with X, and a negative correlation means that Y decreases linearly as X increases. Zero correlation reflects a complete non-association between the compared variables. When a researcher checks relationship between two variables it is very true that the causation always implies correlation but correlation does not necessarily imply causation.

TYPES OF CORRELATION (FIG. 19.1)

Correlation is classified into various types.
- Positive and negative correlation
- Linear and non-linear correlation

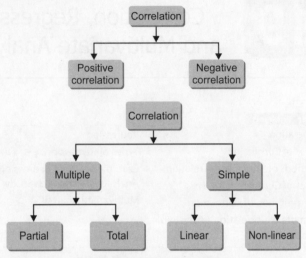

Figure 19.1: Types of correlation.

- Partial and total correlation
- Simple and multiple correlations.

Positive correlation: The correlation is said to be a positive correlation if the values of the two variables changing in the same direction. That is if one increases the other one also increases; if one decreases the other one also decreases, e.g. Height and weight.

Negative correlation: The correlation is said to be a negative correlation when the values of the two variables change with opposite direction, e.g. Disability and quality of life.

Simple correlation: In this only relationship between two variables are studied (Bivariate).

Multiple correlations: Where relationship between three or more than three variables are studied.

Partial correlation: Analysis recognizes more than two variables but considers only two variables keeping the other constant.

Total correlation: It is based on all the relevant variables of the research objective.

Linear correlation: Correlation is said to be linear when the amount of change in one variable tends to bear a constant ratio to the amount of change in the other

Non-linear correlation: The correlation would be non-linear if the amount of change in one variable does not bear a constant ratio to the amount of change in the other variable.

METHODS OF STUDYING CORRELATION

1. **Scatter diagram:** It is the simplest method of studying the relationship between two variables diagrammatically. One variable is represented along the horizontal axis and the second variable along the vertical axis. For each pair of observations of two variables, we put a dot in the plane. There are as many dots in the plane as the number of paired observations of two variables. The direction of dots shows the scatter or concentration of various points. This will show the type of correlation (Fig. 19.2).

2. **Correlation co-efficient:** The degree of relationship between the variables under consideration is a measure through the correlation analysis. The measure of correlation is called as the correlation coefficient. Usually the degree of relationship is expressed by correlation coefficient ranges from $(-1 \leq r \geq +1)$. The correlation analysis enable us to have an idea about the degree and direction of the relationship between the two variables considered by the researcher. The correlation co-efficient is usually presented with appropriate p-values and confidence intervals. The correlation coefficient is also used as an indicator of prediction. If a strong positive or negative correlation is obtained, then the relationship between the two variables may be considered to a predictive relationship.

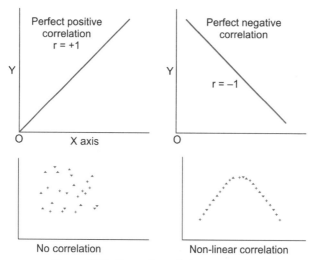

Figure 19.2: Types of correlation scatter plot.

```
I------------------I------------------I------------------I------------------I
-1.0            -0.5               0              +0.5               +1.0
strong negative              no relationship           strong positive
 relationship                                            relationship
```

TYPES OF CORRELATION ANALYSIS

Coefficient of correlation 'r' primarily measures the strength and direction of linear relationship between two variables.

1. Karl Pearson's r: A measure of the strength of a relationship between two continuous variables, e.g. Range of motion of knee and speed of gait.
2. Spearman's Rho: A measure of the similarity between two ordinal rankings of a single set of data, e.g. Grades of spasticity before and after treatment.
3. Point-Biserial r: A measure of the strength of a relationship between one continuous variable and one dichotomous variable, e.g. Yes or No; gender.
4. Phi (ϕ) correlation: A measure of the strength of a relationship between two dichotomous or binary variables, e.g. Gender (male/female) and satisfaction (yes/no). This is similar to the Pearson correlation coefficient in its interpretation.

1. Karl Pearson's correlation co-efficient (r)

$$r = \frac{\Sigma(x-\bar{x})(y-\bar{y})}{\sqrt{\Sigma(x-\bar{x})^2(y-\bar{y})^2}}$$

It summarizes in one value, the degree of correlation and direction of correlation also.

Assumptions for **correlation analysis:**

a. Related data pairs or repeated measure data: Same participants must provide the scores of both the variables, e.g. test-retest scores for a reliability study.
b. Numerical data: Ratio or interval data.
c. Normality: The scores must be normally distributed.
d. Linearity: A linear relationship.
e. Homoscedasticity: Variability in one variable is approximately same at all values of the other variable.

f. Outliers in the data should be kept to a minimum or are removed entirely.

When the above mentioned assumptions are not met the non-parametric Spearman's rank order correlation can be used.

The effect size criteria for interpretation of Pearson correlation coefficient is 0.1 = small; 0.3 = medium and .5 = large.

2. **Spearman's rank correlation co-efficient (p)**

$$p = 1 - \frac{6\Sigma d^2}{n^3 - 3}$$

This method is used where the data are in the form of ranks.

INTERPRETATION OF CORRELATION

A very small correlation does not necessarily indicate that two variables are not associated because it is possible that the two variables display a non-linear relationship. In such cases r will underestimate the association, as it is a measure of linear association alone.

Solution: Do consider transforming the data to obtain a linear relation before calculating r.

Very small r values may be statistically significant in moderately large samples. The calculation $100r^2$ (the coefficient of determination), which is the percentage of variability in the data that is 'explained' by the association. So a correlation of 0.8 implies that just about half (64%) of the variability may be put down to the observed association. Table 19.1 lists the qualitative description and strength of correlation coefficient between +1 and –1.

Table 19.1: Strength of correlation

Qualitative description of the strength of correlation coefficient	Evans (1996) suggests effect sizes for the absolute value of r:
–1 perfect negative	.00-.19 "very weak"
(–1, –0.75) strong negative	.20-.39 "weak"
(–0.75, –0.5) moderate negative	.40-.59 "moderate"
(–0.5, –0.25) weak negative	.60-.79 "strong"
(–0.25, 0.25) no linear association	.80-1.0 "very strong"
(0.25, 0.5) weak positive	
(0.5, 0.75) moderate positive	
(0.75, 1) strong positive	
1 perfect positive	

EXAMPLE OF CORRELATION ANALYSIS IN A RESEARCH STUDY

Table19.2: Correlation analysis in a research study

	1	2	3	4	5	6	7	8	9	10
1. Age	1.000	.027	-.404**	-.430**	-.374**	-.440**	-.113	.169**	-.072	.168**
2. Type of work		1.000	.135*	.170**	.129*	.093	.048	-.118	-.102	-.133*
3. HTN			1.000	.305**	.654**	.287**	.083	-.208**	.084	-.159**
4. Body pain				1.000	.333**	.422**	.120	-.269**	.017	-.158**
5. Medica-tion					1.000	.301**	-.001	-.186**	.114	-.132*
6. SF12PCS						1.000	.079	-.286**	.164**	-.230**
7. SF12MCS							1.000	-.485**	-.067	-.145*
8. IWQoL								1.000	.001	.276**
9. IPAQ									1.000	-.136*
10. BMI										1.000

**Correlation is significant at the 0.01 level (2-tailed)
*Correlation is significant at the 0.05 level (2-tailed).

The above table shows the correlation between BMI and HRQoL and its association with demographic and health characteristics of subjects. More age, white collar work type, HTN, body pain, medication were related to increased BMI (coding 1-yes; 2-No). Moreover more BMI had negative correlation with physical component score (PCS) and mental component score (MCS) of HRQoL. Subjects with increased BMI also had low physical activity and positive correlation to impact of weight on quality of life (IWQoL) total score. The PCS and MCS scores were negatively related to IWQoL scores.

REGRESSION

Regression is the measure of the average relationship between two or more variables in terms of the original units of the data. After knowing the relationship between two variables we may be interested in estimating (predicting) the value of one variable given the value of another. The variable predicted on the basis of other variables is called the "dependent" or the 'explained' variable and the other the 'independent' or the 'predicting' variable. Regression analysis provides estimates of values of the dependent variables from the values of independent variables.

TYPES OF REGRESSION

The regression analysis can be classified into:

a. Simple and multiple regressions: The simple or bivariate linear regression model is designed to study the relationship between a pair of variables that appear in a data set. The multiple linear regression model is designed to study the relationship between one variable and several of other variables.

b. Linear and non-linear regression: Linear regression model is designed to study the relationship between the variables which are linearly related that is change in one variable constantly make change in the other one. But in non-linear it is not a constant change even though there is a relationship between them, e.g. curve linear relationship.

c. Total and partial regression: Partial regression is used in multiple linear regression analysis in which the dependent variable increases when one independent variable is increased by one unit and all the other independent variables are held constant. But in total regression all the independent variables are included in analysis not kept constant.

Assumptions in Regression Analysis

A linear relationship between dependent and independent variables (A scatter plot indicates whether these variables are linearly related).

The dependent variable takes any random value but the values of the independent variables are fixed.

For each value of the independent variable, the distribution of the dependent variable must be normal.

The variance of the distribution of the dependent variable should be constant for all values of the independent variable.

All observations should be independent.

The dependent and independent variables should be quantitative.

Linear Regression Equation

If two variables have linear relationship then as the independent variable (X) changes, the dependent variable (Y) also changes.

For any linear-regression equation of the form $y = \alpha + \beta x + e$ 'y' is referred to as the dependent variable and x as the independent variable, since we are trying to predict y from x. In this case, "α" (the intercept) represents the value of y when x is zero, and "β" is the slope of the regression line. A positive value of β implies that the slope rises from left to right, and a negative value implies that it declines. Confidence intervals can be obtained for the slope and can be fitted around the regression line to give, for example, a 95% confidence interval for the mean value of y for a given value of x. In regression analysis it is important to mention the R^2, which is interpreted as the proportion of the variability in the data explained by regression. The effect of several independent x variables can be evaluated simultaneously using multiple regression equation with the aim of identifying which independent variables are more influential dependent variable.

Example: Body weight is the independent variable and resting heart rate is the dependent variable, since body weight is used to predict the RMR level of individuals.

EXAMPLE OF LINEAR REGRESSION ANALYSIS IN A RESEARCH STUDY (TABLE 19.3)

Table 19.3: Regression analysis of outcomes in a study

Dependent Variable	Independent variable	Adjusted R square %	Constant	Unstandard-ized B	'P' value
Physical health	–	–	–	–	–
Psychological health	Pain	9.2	75.975	–5.590	.011
	Locomotion	12.7	45.126	2.418	.003
Social health	Transfer	10.9	105.645	–6.515	.006
Environmental health	Pain Total joint score	21.9	89.281	–9.543 –.139	.005 .841
	Locomotion	5.6	56.584	1.905	.039
Self-care	–	–	–	–	–
Transfer	Pain Bleeding Total joint score	38.8	7.633	–.056 –.948 –.111	.843 .006 .146
Locomotion	Total joint score	13.3	10.498	–.230	.003
Total functional independence	Pain Bleeding Total joint score	20.1	29.49	.271 –.354 –.443	.716 .687 .030

The above table shows the variability predictor or independent variables on the dependent or criterion variable. For example, the pain component has got 9.2% variability on psychological health and as said earlier the unstandardized B =-5.590 indicates that pain downsizes the psychological health.

MULTIVARIATE ANALYSIS (TABLE 19.4)

It is a type of statistics in which analysis of data with more than one dependent or Y variable is done. In multivariate analysis simultaneous observation and analysis of more than one outcome variable has been carried out. Factor analysis, principal components analysis (PCA), discriminant analysis, canonical analysis and multivariate analysis of variance (MANOVA) are all well-known multivariate analysis techniques.

Factor analysis (FA) is an exploratory technique applied to a set of outcome variables that seeks to find the underlying factors. Factor analysis is carried out on the correlation matrix of the observed variables. A factor is a weighted average of the original variables. Usually the goal of factor analysis is to aid data interpretation and to reduce the interpretation of, say for example, a 30-question test to the study of 4 or 5 factors. Moreover, it provides construct validity evidence of self-reporting scales.

1. Exploratory factor analysis: Used to explore the dimensionality of a measurement instrument by finding the smallest number of interpretable factors.
2. Confirmatory factor analysis: Used to study how well a hypo-thesized factor model fits a new sample from the same population or a sample from a different population.

Principal components analysis is a data analysis tool which is used to reduce the dimensionality or number of variables from a large number of interrelated variables. It calculates an uncorrelated set of variables known as factors or principal components. Moreover, it always yields the same solution from the same data which is not a case in factor analysis.

The primary objectives of factor analysis are:

1. Reduction of number of factors or variables
2. Unidimensionality of constructs evaluation
3. Evaluation of construct validity of the tool
4. Development of theoretical constructs and proving proposed theories
5. Examine the structure or relationship between variables.

Canonical correlation analysis is the study of the linear relationship between two sets of variables. It is the multivariate extension of correlation analysis.

Discriminant analysis is a technique used to find a set of prediction equations based on one or more independent variables.

Cluster analysis is a useful exploratory technique to understand the clumping structure of the study data.

Multivariate Analysis of Variance (or MANOVA) is an extension of ANOVA to the case where there are two or more response variables. MANOVA is designed for the case where you have one or more independent factors (each with two or more levels) and two or more dependent variables.

Table 19.4: Multivariate analysis

Dependent variable	Independent variable	Multivariate technique
	Many continuous variables	Factor analysis, cluster analysis
One categorical variable	Many continuous variables	Discriminant analysis/ logistic regression
One continuous variables	Many continuous variables	Multiple regression analysis
Many continuous variables	Many categorical variable	Multivariate analysis of variance
Many continuous and categorical variables	Many continuous variables	Canonical correlation analysis

FURTHER READING

1. Guyatt G, Walter S, Shannon H, Cook D, Jaenschke R, Heddle N. Basic statistics for clinicians: Correlation and regression. Can Med Assoc J. 1995;152:497–504.
2. Hair J, Anderson R, et al. Multivariate data analysis. New Jersey, Prentice-Hall Inc, 1995a.
3. Thompson B. Exploratory and confirmatory factor analysis: Understanding concepts and applications. Washington, DC, American Psychological Association. 2004.

P VALUE

It is derived from the test statistic. It is defined as the probability of getting a difference at least as big as that observed if the null hypothesis is true. For example, if a therapist thinks that Indian physiotherapists look beautiful among all the therapists in allied health and want to test the hypothesis. A criterion was set as to what is beauty. A research is conducted, and the mean score {"test statistic t"} of Physiotherapists was higher compared to other therapists. Now, in the sample we selected, probability of finding the true mean score for the beauty of physiotherapists is represented p-value. And as the mean score is higher, i.e., most of the sampled therapists are beautiful. Then the selected samples' statistic asks to reject null hypothesis and accept alternative hypothesis. Normally the larger the test statistic (example: t/Z score), the smaller the p value. The p value decreases as the test statistic z gets further away from zero (Fig. 20.1).

$p < 0.5$ means the probability of result by chance is less than one in two.
$p < 0.1$ means the probability of result by chance is less than one in 10.
$p < 0.05$ means the probability of result by chance is less than one in 20.

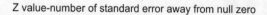

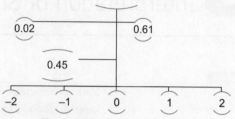

Figure 20.1: P value and z score.

p < 0.025 means the probability of result by chance is less than one in 40.

p < 0.01 means the probability of result by chance is less than one in 100.

p < 0.001 means the probability of result by chance is less than one in 1000.

Normally in physiotherapy research as well as in any health research, 'p < 0.05' is the accepted threshold value for statistical significance. In other words, p < 0.05 represents that there is minimum degree of evidence needed in order to reject the null hypothesis. p-values greater than 0.05 are deemed non-significant, whereas p-values less than 0.05 are deemed statistically significant.

Table 20.1: p value interpretation

p-values less than 0.05	Result is significant	Null hypothesis is rejected
p-values greater than 0.05	Result is non-significant	Null hypothesis cannot be rejected

Even though the p-value shows or reveals strong evidence against the null hypothesis and when it is significant, it is very essential to examine and represent the confidence interval to ascertain whether the range of values for the difference between groups is consistent with the data.

1. In physiotherapy research the probability value less than 5% (p <0.05) is considered as statistically significant result.
2. This cut–off value is arbitrary.
3. It is calculated by a strategy called "hypothesis testing".

CONFIDENCE INTERVAL

A confidence interval (CI) is a **range of values** within which the **true value** lies in. The confidence interval can take any number of probabilities, with the most common being 68%, 95% or 99%.

68% CI = Score ± Standard error

95% CI = Score ± (1.96 × Standard error)

99% CI = Score ± (2.58 × Standard error)

For example, if a researcher is studying the knee ROM after knee joint replacement, he takes a random sample from the population and establishes a mean of 70 degrees. Assuming that the selected sample is normal distribution, by establishing a 95% CI using the sample's mean and standard deviation, the researcher arrives at an upper and lower bound that contains the true mean 95% of the time. Assume that the interval is 65 degrees to 75 degrees. If the researchers take 100 random samples from the population the mean should fall between 65 and 75 degreess in 95 of those samples. If the researchers want even greater confidence, they can expand the interval to 99% confidence. If they establish the 99% CI as 60 degrees to 80 degrees, they can expect 99 of 100 samples evaluated to contain a mean value between these numbers.

Confidence intervals are increasingly preferred than p-values when presenting clinical results. The p-values is about accepting or rejecting the statements we are researching for. The p-values can only reveal whether a result observation is significant or not, but confidence intervals, on the other hand, are far more straightforward as proof statements as presented as a range and offer more information about the properties of a result, i.e. the strength of the statement upon which we accepted the hypothesis. Confidence interval explains the 'clinical importance' of the result findings and its precision.

1. The width of the confidence interval is directly proportional to the level of confidence (99%, 95% or 90%).
2. More the sample size less the width of the confidence interval (i.e. more precise is the result of the study).
3. It is commonly represented in research by graph.
4. Confidence interval is calculated using formulae according to the type of the study data.

Important Points

- The 'p' value is not capable of distinguishing between the absence of evidence of benefit and evidence of absence of benefit (Evidence of absence of benefit means there is enough data to find that the benefit is absent for the intervention. Whereas absence of evidence of benefit means there is no enough data to make a decision about the benefit of the intervention). But the confidence interval can do that.
- The "p" value may not able to distinguish a small effect in a large sample study and a large effect in a small sample study. In both 'p' value may be same.

CLINICAL SIGNIFICANCE AND STATISTICAL SIGNIFICANCE

When a research finding of a study was "**statistically significant**," it does not mean that the findings are important for application in the field. Statistical significance can only reveal whether the differences observed between groups being studied are real or simply due to chance. The statistical hypothesis testing is done using various tests to determine whether the result of a data set in a study is **statistically significant**. The p-value could explain the result (probability of random chance). In general, a p-value of 5% (0.05) or lower is considered to be **statistically significant**.

Clinical significance is the practical importance of a treatment effect - whether it has a real genuine, palpable, noticeable effect on daily life. How effective is the intervention or treatment, or how much change does the treatment cause as effect? It gives quantified information about the importance of a finding, using metrics such as effect size, number needed to treat (NNT), and preventive fraction. The statistical **significance** is often confused with **clinical significance**.

EFFECT SIZE

In research effect size is the magnitude of the difference between groups. In practical terms it is difference between averages, means or any outcomes between two or more intervention groups. It is important to always present effect sizes for primary outcomes. If the units of measurement are meaningful on a practical level (e.g. number of cigarettes smoked per day), then we usually prefer an

unstandardized measure (regression coefficient or mean difference) to a standardized measure (r or d).
— *L. Wilkinson and APA Task Force on Statistical Inference (1999, p.599)*

Effect size is a simple way of quantifying the difference between two groups that has many advantages over the use of tests of statistical significance alone. Effect size emphasizes the size of the difference rather than confounding this with sample size. Moreover Effect sizes complement statistical hypothesis testing, and play an important role in power analyses, sample size planning, and in meta-analyses.

It can be used, for example, to accompany reporting of t-test and ANOVA results. It is also widely used in meta-analysis. Cohen's d is an appropriate effect size for the comparison between two means. Cohen's d is determined by calculating the mean difference between two groups, and then dividing the result by the pooled standard deviation. Cohen's d is the appropriate effect size measure if two groups have similar standard deviations and are of similar size. If Cohen's d is bigger than 1, the difference between the two means is larger than one standard deviation, anything larger than 2 means that the difference is larger than two standard deviation.

The effect size is just the standardized mean difference between the two groups. In other words:

$$\text{Effect size} = \frac{[\text{Mean of experimental group}] - [\text{Mean of control group}]}{\text{Standard Deviation}}$$

An effect size is exactly equivalent to a 'Z-score' of a standard Normal distribution. For example, an effect size of 0.8 means that the score of the average person in the experimental group is 0.8 standard deviations above the average person in the control group.

Alternative Measures of Effect-Size

Cohen's w (for chi square)
Odds ratio
R^2 (regression coefficient)
Risk ratio (RR)
Risk difference (RD)
Rank-biserial correlation (non-parametric man Whitney U)
Cliff's delta (ordinal data)

STANDARD ERROR OF MEASUREMENT

The standard error of measurement (SEM) is a measure of how much measured test scores from different samples are spread around a "true" score in the whole population. It is the repeated measures of a person on the same instrument which tend to be distributed around his or her "true" score. The true score is always an unknown because no measure can be constructed that provides a perfect reflection of the true score.

The formula is:

$$SEM = S\sqrt{1 - r_{xx}}$$

[S-test score standard deviation; r_{xx}-test score reliability]

Standard error of measurement is directly related to a test's reliability: The larger the SEM, the lower the test's reliability.

If test reliability = 0, the SEM will equal the standard deviation of the observed test scores.

If test reliability = 1.00, the SEM is zero.

Table 20.2: Estimates of dispersion

Standard deviation	Estimates the dispersion in a given distribution	Standard deviation* $(\sigma) = \sqrt{\dfrac{\Sigma(X_i - \bar{X})^2}{n}}$ $X_i = i$th values of the variable X n = number of items; $\bar{X}$ = Arithmetic average;
Standard error of the mean	Estimates the dispersion of sampling errors when you are trying to estimate the population mean from a sample mean	$S_M = \dfrac{S}{\sqrt{N}}$ S_M = standard error of the mean S = standard deviation of the mean N = number of scores on the test
Standard error of measurement	Estimates the dispersion of the measurement errors	$SEM = S\sqrt{1 - r_{xx}}$ SEM = standard error of measurement S = standard deviation of the test r_{xx} = reliability of the test
Standard error of estimate	Estimates the dispersion of prediction errors in regression analysis	see $= S_Y\sqrt{1 - r_{yx^2}}$ SEE = standard error of estimate S_Y = standard deviation of the Y values in the original regression analysis r_{yx^2} = correlation squared of Y and X values in the original regression analysis

The standard deviation, standard error of the mean, standard error of measurement, and standard error of estimate are quite different things. They are all based on the simple notions of the normal distribution, but they have quite different applications in research. Table 20.2 describes the definitions and formulae for estimates and related parameters in a research.

MINIMAL DETECTABLE CHANGE

Minimal detectable change (MDC) is defined as the minimal change that falls outside the measurement error in the score of an instrument used to measure a symptom. The formula to calculate Minimal Detectable Change is $1.96 \times \sqrt{2} \times SEM$. The MDC can be interpreted as the magnitude of change below which there is more than a 95% chance that no real change has occurred.

MINIMAL CLINICALLY IMPORTANT DIFFERENCE

Minimal clinically important difference (MCID) represents the smallest amount of change in an outcome that might be considered important by the patient or clinician. Clinical bottom line: The MCID is a published value of change in an instrument that indicates the minimum amount of change required for your patient to feel a difference in the variable you are measuring. The MCID is typically quantified in the units used in the measurement (e.g. If ROM it may be in degrees). The following methods may be used to calculate MCID:

1. **Distribution-based methods:**
Using the one-half standard deviation: A patient improving more than one-half of the outcome score's standard deviation has achieved a minimal clinically important difference.

One standard error of measurement: A change smaller than the standard error of measurement is likely to be the result of measurement error rather than a true observed change. Patients achieving a difference in outcome score of at least one standard error of measurement would have achieved a minimal clinically important difference.

The effect size: An effect size cut off point can be used to define MCID in the same way as the one half standard deviation and the standard error of measurement.

2. **Anchor method**
It is based on patient's response to treatment, after treatment the patients are asked: "Do you feel that you are improved by your

treatment?" Differences between those who favored and unfavored the treatment form the basis of the anchor method.

3. Delphi method

The Delphi method relies on a panel of experts who reach consensus regarding the MCID. The expert panel is provided with information on the results of a trial and are requested to provide their best estimate of the MCID. Their responses are averaged, and this summary is sent back with an invitation to revise their estimates. This process is continued until consensus is achieved.

NUMBER NEEDED TO TREAT

The NNT is the average number of patients who need to be treated to prevent one additional bad outcome (e.g. the number of patients that need to be treated for one of them to benefit compared with a control in a clinical trial). It is defined as the inverse of the absolute risk reduction (1/ARR). The higher the NNT, the less effective is the treatment.

Example:

	Good Outcome	Bad Outcome
Control	59	2
Experimental	61	0

Calculated Results

3.28% of control subjects had the adverse outcome.
0.00% of experimental subjects had the adverse outcome.
The difference, the absolute risk reduction, is 3.28%.

The 95% confidence interval for this difference ranges from -1.19% to 7.75%.

The NNT (Number needed to treat) is 31. This means that about one in every 31 patients will benefit from the treatment. Moreover, the 95% confidence interval for the absolute risk reduction extends from a negative number (treatment may harm) to a positive number (treatment may benefit).

With 95% certainty that one of these statements is true: The experimental treatment is helpful (compared to control), and the number needed to help is greater than 12.9, OR the experimental treatment is harmful (compared to control), and the number needed to harm is greater than 84.0.

EFFICACY

Efficacy refers to the ability of a treatment or intervention to provide a beneficial effect.

Efficacy (therapeutic effect) determines whether an intervention produces the expected result under ideal circumstances. **Effectiveness** measures the degree of beneficial effect under "real world" clinical settings.

The formula is 1-RR (RR- risk ratio).

FURTHER READING

1. Altman D. Practical statistics for medical research. London: Chapman and Hall, 1995:210–2.
2. Attia A. Why should researchers report the confidence interval in modern research? Middle East Fertil Soc J. 2005;10:78-81.
3. Evans SJ, Mills P, Dawson J. The end of the P value? Br Heart J. 1988;60:177-80.
4. Gardner MJ, Altman DG (eds). Statistics with confidence: confidence intervals and statistical guidelines. London: BMJ Books, 1989.
5. Greenhalgh T. How to read a paper: Statistics for the non-statistician. II: Significant relations and their pitfalls. BMJ, 1997;315(7105):422-5.
6. Guyatt G, Jaenschke R, Heddle N, Cook D, Shannon H, Walter S. Basic statistics for clinicians. 2. Interpreting study results: confidence intervals. Can Med Assoc J. 1995;152:169–73.
7. Potter RH. Significance level and confidence interval. J Dent Res. 1994; 73:494-6.

PART 3

Understanding and Publishing Research

- ✦ Evidence-based Physiotherapy
- ✦ Research Proposal
- ✦ Understanding a Research Article
- ✦ Methodology in Research Article
- ✦ Critical Appraisal Tools
- ✦ Critical Appraisal of Clinical Trials
- ✦ Systematic Review and Meta-analysis
- ✦ Journal Club

Evidence-based Physiotherapy

EVIDENCE

"Evidence" in medical science is derived knowledge in accordance with scientific method to either support or counter a scientific theory or hypothesis. Strength of scientific evidence is generally based on the results of statistical analysis and the strength of scientific controls. Such evidence is expected to be empirical evidence that is the information acquired by observation or experimentation.

"The testing of a hypothesis or theory that is objective and in a controlled environment."

EVIDENCE-BASED PRACTICE

The most common definition of Evidence-based practice (EBP) is from Dr David Sackett. EBP is "the conscientious, explicit and judicious use of current best evidence in making decisions about the care of the individual patient. It means integrating individual clinical expertise with the best available external clinical evidence from systematic research." (Sackett D, 1996). EBP is the integration of clinical expertise, patient values, and the best research evidence into the decision making process for patient care. Clinical expertise refers to the clinician's cumulated experience, education and clinical skills. The patient brings to the encounter his or her own personal preferences and unique concerns, expectations, and values. The best research evidence is usually found in clinically relevant research that has been conducted using sound methodology. (Sackett D, 2002)

Evidence-based practice requires new skills of the clinician, including efficient literature searching, and the application of formal rules of evidence in evaluating the clinical literature. While the history

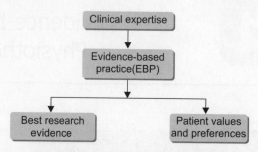

Figure 21.1: Evidence-based practice (EBP).

of EBP stemmed from the main disciplines of medical practice, it is no wonder that the clinical practice of Physiotherapy is slowly getting to adapt and follow the same suit in providing the best care to the beneficiaries – the patients, through evidence base. Thus research forms an important prima fascia upon which the practice of evidence base is dependent on. However more and more empirical research evidences are required in the field of Physiotherapy to follow and implement effective EBP (Fig. 21.1).

Evidence-based practice (EBP) is part of moving clinical practice forward. EBP is required for any clinician to have up to date knowledge to bridge gaps in knowledge, skills and practice to use it in clinical decision making and in turn towards best and efficient patient care. The knowledge that is to be used is dependent of internal and external evidences. Internal evidences are knowledge gathered by the clinician through formal education, clinical practice and clinician-patient relationship. External evidences are information accessible through research. It is the use of valid external evidence combined with the prevailing internal evidence which defines as "evidence-based". For an effective EBP the process involved in turning the evidence that is generated into effective care involves the following five (ASSESS, ASK, ACQUIRE, APPRAISE and APPLY) steps. They form the basis of critically appraised topics or CATs, i.e. appraising of evidence from various research sources.

STEPS IN THE EBP PROCESS

Among the mentioned steps in Table 21.1 the clinicians need to be make themselves skilled in appraisal of the evidence.

The clinical question, which is the starting point of EBP in a specific scenario need to be good to be effective. One method of narrowing the towards an effective question is through PICO method or principle. The construct of PICO is described as follows:

Table 21.1: Steps in the EBP process

ASSESS the patient	1. Start with the patient -- a clinical problem or question arises from the care of the patient
ASK the question	2. Construct a well-built clinical question derived from the case
ACQUIRE the evidence	3. Select the appropriate resource(s) and conduct a search
APPRAISE the evidence	4. Appraise the evidence for its validity (closeness to the truth) and applicability (usefulness in clinical practice)
APPLY: Talk with the patient	5. Return to the patient -- integrate that evidence with clinical expertise, patient preferences and apply it to practice
Self-evaluation	6. Evaluate your performance with this patient

- Anatomy of a good clinical question: PICO
  PICO is a mnemonic that helps one remember the key components of a well-focused question. P = Patient Problem; I = Intervention, prognostic factor or exposure; C = Comparison; O = Outcome.
- Two additional elements of the well-built clinical question are the type of question and the type of study. This information can be helpful in focusing the question and determining the most appropriate type of evidence or study.
  Table 21.2 describes about the examples on the type of questions that may commonly arise in various clinical scenarios and the information to look for from the type of research studies.

Table 21.2: Common type of questions and their study designs

Most common type of questions	Type of study
Diagnosis How to select and interpret diagnostic tests	Prospective, blind comparison to a gold standard or cross-sectional
Therapy How to select treatments that do more good than harm and that are worth the efforts and costs of using them	Randomized controlled trial > cohort study
Prognosis How to estimate the patient's likely clinical course over time (*based on factors other than the intervention*) and anticipate likely complications of disease	Cohort study > case control > case series
Harm/Etiology How to identify causes for disease (including iatrogenic forms)	Cohort > case control > case series

- Choosing the best resource to search is an important decision. Large internet based databases such as PubMed/MEDLINE will give the researcher access to the primary literature. Secondary resources such as ACP Journal Club, Essential Evidence, FPIN Clinical Inquiries, and Clinical Evidence will provide you with an assessment of the original study. The Cochrane Library provides access to systematic reviews which help summarize the results from a number of studies. These are often called "pre-appraised" or EBP resources.

Table 21.3 lists the major professional online databases containing research articles from health services (NHS), respective professional areas like medicine, surgery, pharmacy, physiotherapy, nursing etc., other sources of information like e-books.

Table 21.3: Major professional online databases for evidence search

NHS Evidence	Great place to get the cream of the evidence – searches a limited number of high quality sources.
TRIP database	Great place to get the cream of the evidence – searches a limited number of high quality sources.
Cochrane Library	The source of systematic reviews.
Pubmed Medline	Great starting point for any health or medical literature search.
Embase	Very complementary to Medline with strengths in pharmacology, drug research and toxicology.
CINAHL via NHS ATHENS	Prime source of nursing and allied health literature.
BNI	British Nursing Index – great source of nurse literature.
PsycINFO	Prime source for psychology and psychiatry literature.
Web of Science	Multi-disciplinary database, including links to Citation Indexes (citing articles) and Journal Impact Factors.

Contd...

Contd...

Scopus	Multi-disciplinary database, including links to citing articles.
AMED	Allied and Complementary Medicine Database.
PEDro	Physiotherapy Evidence Database.
OTSeeker	Searches systematic reviews and randomized controlled trials relevant to occupational therapy.
http://www.opengrey.eu/ https://clinicaltrials.gov/ The Trials Register of Promoting Health Interventions (TRoPHI). http://www.who.int/ictrp/en/	Good sources of grey literature
http://annals.org/aim/journal-club http://www.clinicalevidence.bmj.com/ http://www.ebscohost.com/dynamed/aboutUs.php http://www.essentialevidenceplus.com/ http://fpin.org/page/CIOverview http://www.uptodate.com/	EBP Resources
http://accessmedicine.mhmedical.com/ https://www.clinicalkey.com/ http://online.statref.com/Bookshelf. aspx?grpalias=DMCL2	E-Books and Libraries

The Cochrane Library

The Cochrane Library produces world-leading systematic reviews and research on evidence-based health care through seven comprehensive databases. The Cochrane Library provides independent, high-quality, evidence on the latest medical treatments and is designed to facilitate the choices that doctors, patients, policy makers, and others face in health care.

EBM Guidelines

EBM guidelines is an easy-to-use collection of clinical guidelines for primary and ambulatory care linked to the best available evidence.

Evidence-Based Healthcare Books

Wiley-Blackwell continues to develop its wide range of evidence-based textbooks, covering all of the most important medical specialties.

These books use the best evidence to inform treatment decisions for each therapy area.

For more information - www.evidencebasedseries.com

Table 21.4: Physiotherapy journals with open access (for more details :http://physicaltherapyweb.com/physical-therapy-journals/)

1. Australian Journal of Physiotherapy - http://www.physiotherapy.asn.au/index.php/quality-practice/ajp/ajp-archive
2. European Journal of Physical and Rehabilitation Medicine - http://www.minervamedica.it/en/journals/europa-medicophysica/archive.php
3. Journal of Physical Therapy Science - http://www.jstage.jst.go.jp/browse/jpts/_vols
4. Journal of Neurologic Physical Therapy-http://journals.lww.com/jnpt/Pages/issuelist.aspx
5. Journal of Orthopedic & Sports Physical Therapy http://www.jospt.org/issues/type.2/pastissues.asp
6. Physical Therapy Journal - http://ptjournal.apta.org/content/by/year
7. International Journal of Therapies and Rehabilitation Research-http://www.scopemed.org/?mno=19333
8. International Journal of Physiotherapy-http://www.ijphy.org/
9. Indian Journal of Physical Therapy-http://www.indianjournalofphysicaltherapy.in/
10. Journal of Rehabilitation Medicine-http://www.medicaljournals.se/jrm/
11. Journal of Sport Rehabilitation-http://journals.humankinetics.com/jsr
12. Manual Therapy-http://www.manualtherapyjournal.com/
13. New Zealand Journal of Physiotherapy-https://pnz.org.nz/journal
14. Physical Therapy in Sport http://www.physicaltherapyinsport.com/
15. Journal of Biomechanics-http://www.jbiomech.com/

LEVELS OF EVIDENCE

The cornerstone of EBP is the hierarchical system of evidence otherwise known as levels of evidence. Originally developed by Canadian task force on the periodic health examination which was expanded towards a system of rating evidence by Sackett et al in 1989. Initially RCTs were kept at the highest level in evidence pyramid. Further modifications in the levels of evidence were carried out with levels categorized into treatment, diagnosis, prognosis and economic/decision analysis. Currently the five levels of evidence for diagnostic and intervention studies that are defined as follows

Five Levels of Evidence

Level	Research Design	Description
Level 1	Randomized controlled trial (RCT)	Randomized controlled trial, PEDro score 6. Includes within subjects comparison with randomized conditions and cross-over designs
Level 2	RCT	Randomized controlled trial, PEDro score < 6.
	Prospective controlled trial	Prospective controlled trial (not randomized)
	Cohort	Prospective longitudinal study using at least 2 similar groups with one exposed to a particular condition.
Level 3	Case control	A retrospective study comparing conditions, including historical controls
Level 4	Pre-post	A prospective trial with a baseline measure, intervention, and a post-test using a single group of subjects.
	Post-test	A prospective post-test with two or more groups (intervention followed by post-test and no re-test or baseline measurement) using a single group of subjects.
	Case Series	A retrospective study usually collecting variables from a chart review.
Level 5	Observational	Study using cross-sectional analysis to interpret relations.
	Clinical Consensus	Expert opinion without explicit critical appraisal, or based on physiology, biomechanics or "first principles"
	Case Report	Pre-post or case series involving one subject

(Editors: Riegelman, Richard K. Title: Studying a Study and Testing a Test: How to Read the Medical Evidence, 5th Edition, 2005, Lippincott Williams & Wilkins).

As we move up the pyramid the study designs are more rigorous and allow for less bias or systematic error and the information thus gathered from the top of pyramid has higher reliability compared to low level studies.

Case series and Case reports consist of collections of reports on the treatment of individual patients or a report on a single patient on a specific. Because they are reports of cases and use no control groups to compare outcomes, they have little statistical validity.

Case control studies are studies in which patients who already have a specific condition who are compared with people who do not have the condition. The researcher looks back to identify factors or exposures that might be associated with the illness. They often rely on medical records and patient recall for data collection. These types of studies are often less reliable than randomized controlled trials and cohort studies because showing a statistical relationship does not mean than one factor necessarily caused the other (no causal effect).

Cohort studies identify a group of patients who are already taking a particular treatment or have an exposure, follow them forward over time, and then compare their outcomes with a similar group that has not been affected by the treatment or exposure being studied. Cohort studies are observational and not as reliable as randomized controlled studies, since the two groups may differ in ways other than in the variable under study.

Randomized controlled clinical trials are carefully planned experiments that introduce a treatment or exposure to study its effect on real patients. They include methodologies that reduce the potential for bias (randomization and blinding) and that allow for comparison between intervention groups and control (no intervention) groups. A randomized controlled trial is a planned experiment and can provide sound evidence of cause and effect.

Systematic reviews focus on a clinical topic and answer a specific question. An extensive literature search is conducted to identify studies with sound methodology. The studies are reviewed, assessed for quality, and the results summarized according to the predetermined criteria of the review question.

A **Meta-analysis** will thoroughly examine a number of valid studies on a topic and mathematically combine the results using accepted statistical methodology to report the results as if it were one large study.

Cross-sectional studies describe the relationship between diseases and other factors at one point in time in a defined population. Cross sectional studies lack any information on timing of exposure and outcome relationships and include only prevalent cases. They are often used for comparing diagnostic tests. Studies that show the efficacy of a diagnostic test are also called **prospective, blind comparison to a gold standard** study. This is a controlled trial that looks at patients with varying degrees of an illness and administers both diagnostic tests — the test under investigation and the "gold standard" test — to all of the patients in the study group. The sensitivity and specificity of the new test are compared to that of the gold standard to determine potential usefulness.

Retrospective cohort (or historical cohort) follows the same direc tion of inquiry as a cohort study. Subjects begin with the presence or absence of an exposure or risk factor and are followed until the outcome of interest is observed. However, this study design uses information that has been collected in the past and kept in files or databases. Patients are identified for exposure or non-exposures and the data is followed forward to an effect or outcome of interest.

COMMONLY USED EVIDENCE RATING SCALES

There are different scales available from major centers promoting evidence-based practice of various countries to evaluate and rate the level of evidences. Few are mentioned here:

Centre for Evidence-Based Medicine, Oxford-levels (1a-5)
SORT: Strength-of-Recommendation Taxonomy-levels (A,B,C)
GRADE: Grading of Recommendations Assessment, Development and Evaluation-levels (A,B,C,D)
Practice Guidelines rating scales (various levels).

1. Centre for Evidence-Based Medicine, Oxford (For Therapy/Prevention/Etiology/Harm).

1a: Systematic reviews (with homogeneity) of randomized controlled trials.

1b: Individual randomized controlled trials (with narrow confidence interval).

1c: All or none randomized controlled trials.

2a: Systematic reviews (with homogeneity) of cohort studies.

2b: Individual cohort study or low quality randomized controlled trials (e.g. <80% follow-up).

2c: "Outcomes" Research; ecological studies.

3a: Systematic review (with homogeneity) of case-control studies.

3b: Individual case-control study.

4: Case-series (and poor quality cohort and case-control studies).

5: Expert opinion without explicit critical appraisal, or based on physiology, bench research or "first principles."

Centre for Evidence-Based Medicine, Oxford
Diagnosis

1a: Systematic review (with homogeneity) of Level 1 diagnostic studies; or a clinical decision rule with 1b studies from different clinical centers.

1b: Validating cohort study with good reference standards; or clinical decision rule tested within one clinical center.

1c: Absolute SpPins And SnNouts (An Absolute SpPin is a diagnostic finding whose Specificity is so high that a Positive result rules-in the diagnosis. An Absolute SnNout is a diagnostic finding whose Sensitivity is so high that a Negative result rules-out the diagnosis).

2a: Systematic review (with homogeneity) of Level >2 diagnostic studies.

2b: Exploratory cohort study with good reference standards; clinical decision rule after derivation, or validated only on split-sample or databases.

3a: Systematic review (with homogeneity) of 3b and better studies.

3b: Non-consecutive study; or without consistently applied reference standards.

4: Case-control study, poor or non-independent reference standard.

5: Expert opinion without explicit critical appraisal, or based on physiology, bench research or "first principles."

Centre for Evidence-Based Medicine, Oxford
Prognosis

1a: Systematic review (with homogeneity) of inception cohort studies; or a clinical decision rule validated in different populations.

1b: Individual inception cohort study with > 80% follow-up; or a clinical decision rule validated on a single population.

1c: All or none case-series.

2a: Systematic review (with homogeneity) of either retrospective cohort studies or untreated control groups in randomized controlled trials.

2b: Retrospective cohort study or follow-up of untreated control patients in a randomized controlled trial; or derivation of a clinical decision rule or validated on split-sample only.

2c: "Outcomes" research.

3: None.

4: Case-series (and poor quality prognostic cohort studies).

5: Expert opinion without explicit critical appraisal, or based on physiology, bench research or "first principles."

Note: A minus sign "-" may be added to denote evidence that fails to provide a conclusive answer because it is *either* (a) a single result with a wide Confidence Interval; *OR* (b) a Systematic Review with troublesome heterogeneity. Such evidence is inconclusive, and therefore can only generate Grade D recommendations.

Strength-of-Recommendation Taxonomy (SORT)
Code-Definition
A-Consistent, good-quality patient-oriented evidence*
B-Inconsistent or limited-quality patient-oriented evidence*
C-Consensus, disease-oriented evidence*, usual practice, expert opinion, or case series for studies of diagnosis, treatment, prevention, or screening

* *Patient-oriented evidence measures outcomes that matter to patients: morbidity, mortality, symptom improvement, cost reduction, and quality of life. Disease-oriented evidence measures immediate, physiologic, or*
surrogate end points that may or may not reflect improvements in patient outcomes (e.g. blood pressure, blood chemistry, physiologic function, pathologic findings).

Grading of Recommendations Assessment, Development and Evaluation (GRADE)
Code-Quality of Evidence Definition
A-High
Further research is very unlikely to change our confidence in the estimate of effect.
Several high-quality studies with consistent results.
In special cases: one large, high-quality multi-center trial.

B-Moderate
Further research is likely to have an important impact on our confidence in the estimate of effect and may change the estimate.
One high-quality study.
Several studies with some limitations.

C-Low
Further research is very likely to have an important impact on our confidence in the estimate of effect and is likely to change the estimate.

One or more studies with severe limitations.

D Very Low

Any estimate of effect is very uncertain.

Expert opinion.

No direct research evidence.

One or more studies with very severe limitations.

Source: GRADE (Grading of Recommendations Assessment, Development and Evaluation) Working Group 2007.

Key to Interpretation of Practice Guidelines

Agency for Healthcare Research and Quality

A: There is good research-based evidence to support the recommendation.

B: There is fair research-based evidence to support the recommendation.

C: The recommendation is based on expert opinion and panel consensus.

X: There is evidence of harm from this intervention.

USPSTF Guide to Clinical Preventive Services

A: There is good evidence to support the recommendation that the condition be specifically considered in a periodic health examination.

B: There is fair evidence to support the recommendation that the condition be specifically considered in a periodic health examination.

C: There is insufficient evidence to recommend for or against the inclusion of the condition in a periodic health examination, but recommendations may be made on other grounds.

D: There is fair evidence to support the recommendation that the condition be excluded from consideration in a periodic health examination.

E: There is good evidence to support the recommendation that the condition be excluded from consideration in a periodic health examination.

University of Michigan Practice Guideline

A: Randomized controlled trials.

B: Controlled trials, no randomization.

C: Observational trials.

D: Opinion of the expert panel.

Other Guidelines

A: There is good research-based evidence to support the recommendation.

B: There is fair research-based evidence to support the recommendation.

C: The recommendation is based on expert opinion and panel consensus.

X: There is evidence that the intervention is harmful.

FURTHER READING

1. Greenhalgh T. How to Read a Paper: The Basics of Evidence-Based Medicine: Wiley; 2014.
2. Heneghan C, Badenoch D. Evidence-Based Medicine Toolkit, 2nd Ed.Wiley Blackwell, 2006.
3. Sackett DL, Richardson WS, Rosenberg WMC, Haynes RB. Evidence-based medicine: how to practice and teach EBM. London: Churchill-Livingstone, 1996.
4. Straus SE, et al. Evidence-Based Medicine: How to Practice and Teach EBM.Churchill Livingstone, 2010.

Research Proposal

RESEARCH PROPOSAL

A research proposal is a document proposing a research project and is a concise and coherent summary of the proposed research. The proposal should include an outline of the research objectives or hypothesis and a brief account of prior research in the topic area. The research proposal outlines the process from beginning to end and may be used to request financing needed for the project. The prime purpose of the research proposal is to assess the quality and originality of the ideas, and feasibility of the research project. The research proposal should discuss concisely the whole process involved in planned research starting from problem statement, research methodology, research activities and a time schedule. This brief proposal in a format specific to each institution should be presented to the committee or organization overseeing the research in the institution. However format of research proposal is almost similar in most institutions with minor variations. The next section discuss in detail about the format of research proposal.

RESEARCH PROPOSAL FORMAT (FIG. 22.1)

1. Forwarding form (one page)

It could be a form of one page and it may include the following details: Name of the proposal/project, Study team composition, Name of the institution, Budget of the study, Duration of the study and Study guide. This would be submitted to the research coordinator for approval of doing the research. Further to this, the actual proposal needs to be submitted.

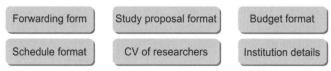

Figure 22.1: Research proposal format.

2. Study proposal

Introduction: Enumerate the details briefly within 100 words. It may include the scientific and technical background of the research title. Literature review on the subject of the study with bibliography (Facts, Concepts, Theories, Previous research findings, Books, journals, reports ,Unpublished data)

Statement of the problem: Enumerate within 100 words (PICO format – if applicable)

Relevance and need of the study: Significance of doing the study- Enumerate within 100 words

Objectives: Purpose of the study-Enumerate within 100 words

Inclusion and exclusion criteria

Definitions-Assumptions-Limitations-Delimitations

Hypothesis

Null hypothesis-alternate hypothesis

Methods

Research design -Sample design-Observational design - type and method-Operational design-Statistical design

(Details of subjects, Tools, Instruments/Equipment, Procedure and Data collection)

Analysis

Planned Qualitative analysis-Quantitative analysis-Statistical test/s used-software used for analysis

Future application of the research -Enumerate within 100 words

Relevant references

Use bibliography cards

3. Schedule format

Duration-plan the number of days/weeks/months required for ground work, planning and execution of the study or simply a time-table about the proceeds of the research.

Example

Subject selection - 4 weeks

Preparation of the tool - 2 weeks

Psychometric validity - 1 month
Pilot study-1 month
Data collection - 6 months
Data analysis - 2 months
Start and end date of the project –March 2017-November 2018.

4. Budget format
Include all the possible expenditure like any-travel expense for the subjects involved in the study, stationary, equipment, preparation of tool, cost of investigations, etc.
For students whether it may be a self-financed or sponsored.

5. Curriculum vitae of the principal and co-investigators
Name of all participants and details .

6. Brief of the institution
Enumerate the details of the institution where research is going to be conducted and facilities in the institution.

7. Endorsement from the head of institution
Prepare a form like format for acceptance of the proposed research by the head of the institution.

PRINCIPLES OF RESEARCH PROPOSAL

Writing a research proposal depends on the purpose and background of the study and is up to the researcher to address the important criteria to simplify the approval process. Even though there is no fixed guidelines the researchers may concentrate on the following principles in their preparation of research proposal.

Background of the research: The question and why the research is important.

How the research is done: When, where and what is done in the study.

Time frame and schedule of the study: Start and finish constraints and deadlines of stages of the study.

Methodology: Way of selecting, allocating and collecting data from participants.

Ethical issues: Informed consent, voluntary participation of subjects.

Data protection: How to ensure confidentiality and anonymity of data.

Dissemination: How the research information will be used or presented.

SAMPLE RESEARCH PROPOSALS

Given below are some sample research proposals involving various study designs.

Example 1: Research proposal for a cross-sectional study.

Title

Quality of life, level of physical activity and depression in dialysis patients: a cross-sectional study.

Researchers

Type name, title, designation, associated institutional address and email id.
Name of the Institution: Sarvajanik College of Physiotherapy.
Year of Research: 2012 – 2013.

Introduction

The increasing prevalence of chronic kidney disease (CKD) has become an international health issue and has drawn much attention worldwide (1). Over the past few decades, quality of life (QOL) (2) research endpoints have emerged as valuable research tools in assessing the outcome of therapeutic intervention in chronic diseases (3). ---
----

Problem Statement/Need and Significance of the Study

It is given that Dialysis is both life-saving and life-altering, however it changes patients' eating, sleeping, medication use, and daily activities at home and in the community. Dialysis and associated symptoms can reduce the ability to work. Therefore we are interested to check effectiveness and outcome of dialysis management. Current study aims to assess the quality of life and psychosocial variables of adult patients in Surat.

Recent studies have suggested that a poor health-related quality of life (HRQOL) is strongly related to increased risk of mortality in patients on dialysis (9 – 15). Thus, although HRQOL is typically used to gain information about patient well-being, it may also indicate the risk of important outcomes, like death.

Purpose of Study

The main objectives of our study are to assess the QOL in hemodialysis patients with reference to their physical, psychological, social, and environmental health dimensions, and to assess the effects of age, sex, income, and level of education, duration of disease, co-morbidity, and treatment duration on the QOL of hemodialysis patients.

Hypothesis

Hypothesis: Mental health of dialysis patient is related to their QOL.
Null hypothesis: There is no relation between depression and QOL of dialysis patients.

Alternate hypothesis: There is a relation between depression and QOL of dialysis patients. --
----

Limitations of the Study

Socio-economic strata/background of patients is not taken into consideration.

The study is a single center one. A very small sample size with less generalizability.

Methods

Study design: Cross-sectional study
Sampling method: Non-probability sampling
Sample size: 100.

Inclusion Criteria:
• Patients on dialysis, above 18 years of age.-------------------------

Exclusion Criteria:
• Progressive neuromuscular disease that may result in limitations
• Orthopedic or rheumatologic disease that may be exacerbated by physical function testing ---

Tools:
• WHO BREF- Questionnaire.
The WHOQOL-BREF consists of 24 facets and provides a profile of scores on four dimensions of quality of life: physical health, psychological, social relationships, and the environment. WHOQOL-BREF is available in both self-administered and interviewer-administered forms. The WHOQOL-BREF questionnaire is available in 19 different languages.(19)

- Beck depression inventory scale.
  The Beck Depression Inventory (BDI) is a series of questions developed to measure the intensity, severity, and depth of depression in patients with psychiatric diagnoses. Its long form is composed of 21 questions, each designed to assess a specific symptom common among people with depression. The BDI has been extensively tested for content validity, concurrent validity, and construct validity. The BDI has content validity because it was constructed from a consensus among clinicians about depressive symptoms displayed by psychiatric patients. For people who have been clinically diagnosed, scores from 0 to 9 represent minimal depressive symptoms, scores of 10 to 16 indicate mild depression, scores of 17 to 29 indicate moderate depression, and scores of 30 to 63 indicate severe depression. (18)---
  ----

Procedure

Patients are taken from dialysis center of XXXX hospital, Surat according to our inclusion and exclusion criteria and are ready to sign consent form to participate in our study. During the study, participants are given questionnaire to complete. Data is collected from each subject and documented in a suitably designed data collection form.

Statistical Analysis

Data will be checked for plausibility and cleaned. Normality of the data will be checked by shaipro -wilk test. Descriptive and exploratory data analysis will be performed on the total data set collected which may include parametric/non parametric tests, chi-square tests, correlation coefficients and linear regression analyses.

Conclusion

The study findings will provide informations about QOL in hemo-dialysis patients with reference to their physical, psychological, social, and environmental health dimensions.

References

1. Dirks JH, de Zeeuw D, Agarwal SK, et al. Prevention of chronic kidney and vascular disease: toward global health equity—the Bellagio 2004 Declaration. Kidney Int Suppl 2005:S1–S6.

2. Beck AT, Steer RA. Internal consistencies of the original and revised Beck Depression Inventory. Journal of Clinical Psychology 40 (1984): 1365-67.
3. Kimmel PL, Peterson RA, Weihs KL, et al. Psychosocial factors, behavioral compliance and survival in urban hemodialysis patients. Kidney Int. 1998;54:245–54.------------------------------
----

Example 2: Research proposal for a reliability and validity study.

Title

Cross-cultural adaptation and psychometric testing of shoulder pain and disability index (SPADI) in Tamil population.

Principal Investigators
Co-investigators
Type name, title, designation, associated institutional address and email id

Background

Shoulder pain is a very common musculoskeletal complaint in middle and old aged populations worldwide, often leading to activity limitations, restricted participation, and thus reduced quality of life [1]. Shoulder pain is defined as, "pain in shoulder with or without pain referred into one or both upper limbs [2] --------------------------
----

Objectives

1. To translate and adapt the shoulder pain and disability index (SPADI) questionnaire cross-culturally in Tamil speaking population.
2. To evaluate feasibility and acceptability; and to estimate internal consistency, test retest reliability, factorial and convergent construct validity.

Methods

Objective 1: *Translation and cross-cultural adaptation*

Protocol

Before translating the SPADI into Tamil language, formal permission will be obtained from the author who had developed the questionnaire. The cross-cultural adaptation process recommended by Beaton et al [13], which includes stages of forward translation, synthesis, back translation, expert committee review, pretesting and appraisal of written reports by the committee will be followed.

In stage 1, two independent translators whose mother tongue is Tamil will do the forward translations (T1 and T2) of the questionnaire in the target language. Each of them will produce individual written reports on their translations. --
----

As the last stage, all written reports will be submitted to the expert committee for proper documentation and future references on the translation process.

Objective 2: *Feasibility, acceptability, factorial validity, internal consistency, test-retest reliability, and construct convergent validity of Tamil SPADI.*

Study Design

A hospital based clinical measurement study with repeated measures design.

Priori Hypotheses

1. The Tamil version of the SPADI questionnaire will demonstrate high internal consistency with Cronbach's alpha >0.7, and test-retest reliability with ICC>0.9.
2. The Tamil SPADI will demonstrate one factor structure with Eigen value above 1
3. The SPADI scores will have moderate to strong correlations ('r' between 0.4 and 0.89) with neck flexion and extension motion ranges, and perceived levels of neck pain and disability.

----

244 Essentials of Research Methodology

Study Participants

Men and women aged between 30-60 years, having neck pain > 1 month, with or without radiating pain and attending the participating the outpatient physiotherapy center in hosmed hospital in Madurai, India will be included.

People will be excluded if they present with rheumatoid arthritis, osteoarthritis, or neck metastases; unable to understand and read Tamil, or unwilling to provide signed consent.

Sample Size

A convenient sample of 155 participants will be included for validity testing, of which 30 will be considered for test-retest reliability evaluation.

Instruments

1. *Shoulder pain and diability Index (Tamil version)*
   Shoulder pain and disability Index [8]
2. *Visual Analogue Scale (Tamil version).*

The VAS [24] will be used to measure patient reported levels of pain intensity and disability in performing their ADL. The VAS for pain is a simple 100 mm horizontal line with anchoring descriptors, 0 for 'no pain' and 100 for 'worst imaginable pain'.

Protocol

Ethics approval for the study protocol will be obtained from the institutional ethics review board, xxxxxx, Madurai. Study recruitment posters will also be posted in several patient waiting areas of the hospital. The staff will directly contact the interested volunteers, screen them for participation criteria, and recruit the eligible volunteers in a consecutive manner. All of the volunteers will be informed of the study purposes and signed consent will be obtained from each of them before evaluation.

After the informed consent process, demographic and clinical information of the study participants will be collected. Clear instructions will be provided on how to complete the paper based

questionnaire and participants will be encouraged to ask questions they might have. --
----

For feasibility evaluation, the time taken to complete the questionnaire will be recorded. For acceptability, percentage of total unanswered questions will be presented.

Statistical Analyses

1. Demographic and clinical information of the study participants will be presented as counts, percentages or means and standard deviations appropriately.
2. Relative test-retest reliability will be determined by Intraclass correlation co-efficient [ICC (2, 1)]. ICC values will be interpreted [1] as very high (ICC>0.9), high (ICC > 0.75), moderate (ICC between 0.5- 0.75) and low (ICC < 0.5) [25].
3. Absolute reliability will be determined by standard error of measurement (SEM) using the formula $SEM = SD \times \sqrt{1 - ICC}$, where SD is the average standard deviation of the two session scores [26, 27, 28]. The minimal detectable change will be calculated using the formula $1.96 \times \sqrt{2} \times SEM$. [27, 28]
4. The limits of agreement between two session scores will be evaluated by plotting the difference in scores during the two testing occasions against the baseline scores in Bland-Altman graph [30, 31].
5. Construct convergent validity will be analyzed using Pearson correlation co-efficient ('r') to determine the strength of the relationship between scores of neck flexion and extension range of motions, VAS pain and disability in ADL. The strength of correlation will be interpreted as .00 to .19-very weak, .20 to .39-weak, .40 to .69-moderate, .70 to .89-strong correlation, and .90 to 1.00-very strong correlation [32].
6. Data will be analyzed using IBM SPSS Statistics for Windows, Version 22.0. Armonk, NY: IBM Corp. A p value of <0.05 (two tailed) will be considered statistically significant.

Conclusions

Findings from this study will provide initial evidence on cross-cultural adaptation process and psychometric properties of SPADI questionnaire in Tamil speaking individuals diagnosed with shoulder pain. Making reliable and valid outcome measures available in Tamil language would help implementing them in clinical practice and research by the health professionals.

References

Mention the references here -------------------------------------

Example 3: Research proposal for an experimental study.
The effectiveness of mechanical cervical traction on mechanical neck pain patients.

Principal Investigators

Co-investigators

Type name, title, designation, associated institutional address and email id

Introduction

Mechanical neck pain (MNP) is also referred to as non-specific neck pain, and is common in all agegroups of people above 18 years of age. It may include discogenic pain, myofascial trigger points, ligaments in the cervical spine; cervical facet syndrome or poor posture may also contribute to this pain. The etiology of neck pain is multifactorial and poorly understood (1) (2). ---------------------------
----
--Gatterman (1990) defines spinal traction as the application of a drawing or a pulling force along the long axis of the spine in order to stretch the soft tissues, separate joint surfaces, to separate bony segments (9)---
----

Need and Significance of the Study

There are many physiotherapy interventions such as Mechanical cervical traction (MCT), mobilization, therapeutic modalities and exercises in neck pain management. There is no comparative study done to find out the effectiveness of the 'MCT with conventional physiotherapy' versus 'conventional physiotherapy alone'.

Purpose of the Study

The aim of the study is to compare the efficacy of 'MCT with conventional physiotherapy' and 'conventional physiotherapy alone' in mechanical neck pain.

Hypothesis

Hypothesis: There is change in the pain scores after the interventions. Null hypothesis: There is no difference between the mean pain score of 'MCT with conventional physiotherapy' and 'conventional physiotherapy alone' in mechanical neck pain patients.

Alternate hypothesis: There is difference between the mean pain score of 'MCT with conventional physiotherapy' and 'conventional physiotherapy alone' in mechanical neck pain patients.

Methods

Design: A randomized controlled clinical trial.

Sampling: Probability sampling.

Sample size: 60.

Inclusion Criteria

Neck pain of less than 4 weeks duration

Numerical pain rating scale (0-10) scores between 4 to 9 to ensure group homogeneity.

The diagnosis of MNP was made using the following criteria : Two of the following three tests had to be present:

1. Kemp's test
2. Cervical compression test
3. Lateral compression test.

Exclusion Criteria

- Neck pain that was not of mechanical origin (13).
- Patients with recent major trauma.

Tools

- Disability of arm, shoulder and hand questionnaire (DASH) (16)
- Numerical pain rating scale (NPRS)
- Cervical spine Goniometry.

Procedure

The participant will be randomly allocated via using a computer generated random allocation table into one of two groups; group A: MCT with conventional therapy, group B: Conventional therapy alone.

Treatment

Group A: MCT with conventional therapy.

Group A: MCT will be given with a motorized traction machine in the form of intermittent traction for 20 minutes with hold time 40 seconds and rest time 10 seconds in supine position with 15° of neck flexion. The pull of traction was 1/10th of subject's body weight.

The conventional therapy includes Ultrasound and Isometric neck exercises. For Ultrasound, position of the participant will be in sitting with head support. Participants will be treated with Ultrasound 1.5 Watt/cm^2 for 8 minutes in continuous mode. For Isometric neck exercises, position of the participant will be in sitting and therapist will stand behind the patient. Isometric neck exercises are applied with 15 repetitions for each of flexion, extension, lateral flexion and cervical rotation with 5 seconds of hold time.

Group B: Conventional therapy alone.

Data Analysis

A repeated measure ANOVA will be used as primary statistical analysis for within-group comparisons. Between-group differences at each follow-up period would be investigated with unpaired t-tests and within group with paired t-test. For the total group correlation analysis will be done. Statistical significance was set at $p < 0.05$ for all statistical analyses. Shapiro-Wilk test will be used to check the normality and all the data analysis will be done in IBM SPSS version 20.0, Armonk, NY: IBM Corp. A p value of < 0.05 (two tailed) will be considered statistically significant.

Conclusion

The findings of the study will provide whether there is any therapeutic effects for cervical traction and if any how much the effectiveness of Mechanical Cervical Traction on Mechanical Neck Pain patients.

References

Mention the references here ------------------------------------

FURTHER READING

1. Al-Riyami A. How to prepare a research proposal. Oman Medical Journal. 2008;23(2):66-69.
2. Pajares F. Elements of proposal 2007. From http://www.des.emory.edu/mfp/proposal.html Accessed June 18, 2008.
3. Wong P. How to write research proposal. International network on Personal meaning. Available at www.meaning.ca/archives Accessed June 18, 2008.

Understanding a Research Article

RESEARCH ARTICLE

It is scientific evidence produced by a researcher or group of researchers to prove some hypotheses or disprove an existing theory. When it is presented for an audience of interest it should be in a formally structured one following some standardized principles.

A research paper is a written discussion which is based on analysis and supported by a collection of ideas and information. It is a way of presenting ideas and facts you have found through the reading of various materials and presentation of findings from a rigorous scientific experimentation or observation.

TYPES OF RESEARCH ARTICLES

Research articles are of many types based on how and what purpose they have been made. Types of research articles are given in the Box 23.1.

Box 23.1: Types of research articles

Original research article: Information based on original research through collected data
Case reports: Usually of a single case
Technical notes: It describes a specific technique or procedure
Pictorial essay: Teaching article with images
Review: Detailed analysis of recent research on a specific topic
Commentary: Short article with author's personal opinions
Editorial: Often short review or critique of original articles
Letter to the Editor: It is short and on subject of interest to readers

COMPONENTS OF AN ARTICLE

The Usual Sequence of a research article

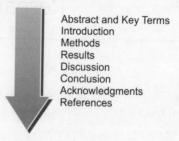

Abstract and Key Terms
Introduction
Methods
Results
Discussion
Conclusion
Acknowledgments
References

Note: Most of the research article publishing journals use a conventional IMRD structure: An abstract followed by Introduction, Methods, Results, and Discussion

Features of Abstract

An abstract is a short and concise statement which details briefly about a large work. Key statements or phrases of the scientific literature are written linking them in an orderly manner which would help readers whether the longer original work is worth their time to read or not. Key statements are usually centered around to highlight the following information.

Abstract usually contain four kinds of information:

1. Purpose or rationale of study (why they did it)
2. Methodology (how they did it)
3. Results (what they found)
4. Conclusion (what it means).

Features of Introduction

Introduction serves two purposes:

1. Creating readers' interest in the subject. Bridge all the relevant information in an order to lead the reader into knowing what and why there is a need for answering the question raised in the research.
2. Providing them with enough information to understand the article.

Features of Methods

The methods section tells the reader what experiments were done, what kind of systematic pathway would be attempted to answer the question.

Features of Results and Discussion

The results section contains results— they are the statements of what was found, and reference to the data shown in visuals (figures and tables). Normally, authors do not include information that would need to be referenced, such as comparison to others' results.

The discussion section provides theoretical analysis based on the results from the research and relate them to the related research information. Analysis informs about the strength and weakness of the current research and how the information generated could be inferred. This would provide a clear answer to the question posed in the Introduction and to explain how the results support that conclusion.

HOW TO READ AN ARTICLE

Every article may not give the necessary outcome of what the reader tries to extract directly or may not be understood by the reader following a casual read. So it is very much important that there should be an in depth plan before getting into this. When a reader tries an attempt to read a research paper, he should plan the following:

1. **What is the way the research paper organized? Is there any difficulty I am going to face?**

Solution: Just superficially skim the article in the first attempt and try to identify the structure of it. Look for poorly written format of the paper, more of jargon in the paper, lack of formal flow, no clear road map, do not clearly distinguish between fact and speculation, overstating the importance of findings (academic frauds).

2. **How can I prepare myself to read a paper, which is a new area of interest to me?**

Solution: Read the title and the abstract first (Most scientists read the abstract first).

The introduction can be skimmed or even skipped (if necessary read the background in a review or textbook).

Read the "Materials and Methods" and "Results" sections multiple times. This would help in better interpretation of the findings.

3. **How do I understand and evaluate the contents of the paper?**

Solution: Try to find out the answers for the following questions which may provide the reader regarding the external validity of the research findings:

- What are the main conclusions of the paper and does evidence and data support those conclusions?

- What is the quality of the evidence?
- Why are the conclusions important?

Actions to be taken while reading a research article
First skim the article without taking notes. Read the "Materials and Methods" and "Results" sections multiple times. Generate questions and be aware of your understanding. Take notes as you read. Draw inferences. Write a draft of your summary.

A CRITICAL REVIEW AND ASSESSMENT OF THE ARTICLE

There are specific things that a researcher should keep in mind before evaluating or reviewing a research paper.

- The reader should include a summary of own analysis and evaluation of the article.
- The reader should know the article thoroughly and avoid personal opinions.
- The reader should focus on the positive aspects of the study learned.
- The reader should note limitations of the study (data not reflecting conclusion, insufficient data, unanswered questions and how can the other researchers improve the study in future).
- The reader may use standardized critical appraisal tools according to the type of the research design the study used.

DUBIOUS DATA IN RESEARCH ARTICLE

A reader should be very careful about the presence of dubious data in the presentation of a research article. It may be in the form of the followings:

Blunders
Sources (who counted and why)
Definitions (what did they count)
Measurements (how did they count)
Packaging (what they are telling)
Rhetoric (what they want us to think)
Debates

The common signs of dubious data presentation in the articles are Slippery decimal points, Botched translations, Misleading graphs, Careless calculations, Big round numbers, Hyperbole (using superlatives), Broad definitions, Odd units of analysis, surrogate end points, Convenient time frames, selective convenient comparisons, misleading samples and statistical adjustments and short-term benefits are converted to long-term benefits.

PRINCIPLES OF WRITING A RESEARCH PAPER

Scientific writing and communication are very important for not only the researchers but also for the publishing to reach its goal. Many of the research results are either not published or rejected by journals because of the poor quality of the writing. The main problems of writing a research article may be in terms of presentation form, substance or content, poor language, improper figures, lack of education and dissemination, cultural differences, results without focus or too many results, without novel findings and communication issues of the writing. The following section may provide a guidance to improve the confidence of scientific writing of researchers.

1. What is a research paper? And why and how does a researcher write a research paper?

   Every research paper is written to find answers to the academic questions which are in due of clinical decision making. A well-written research paper is composed by the use of a variety of outside sources with high credibility. The process of writing requires many steps which are listed in Figure 23.1.

2. Components of a research paper include the parts below:

   Poor or incomplete reporting of information in a research makes many publications of limited value in use for policy making, clinical and scientific practice. Increasingly research communities are directed that the research articles to include relevant information with in-depth critique and highly relevant information. To make sure that reporting are efficient guidelines development was imparted by agencies to improve the quality of reporting. The CONSORT guidelines for RCTs were first developed guidelines followed by other agencies to ensure transparency in reporting research. Other guidelines like EQUATOR, STROBE alike for various types of research design researches were developed. Following components in a research paper are generally accepted as basic by most of the reporting guidelines.

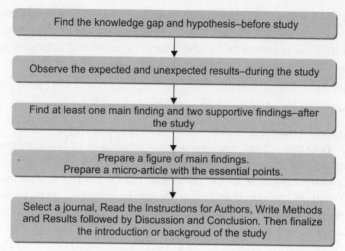

Figure 23.1: Steps for writing a research article.

Title of the research paper
Abstract
Introduction
Literature Review
Methodology
Results
Discussion
Conclusion
References
Appendices

1. Title Page

Choosing a comprehensive title of the study is very important as it is going to make a first impression for the reader to select this for reading.

The title should be written in the middle of the page.

Below the title name(s) of the author(s), the name of the institution and the year of the study should be written.

Somewhere above the title, the running head (as clear and short as possible) should be presented.

The running head should appear on every page with the page number.

Example:
IOSR Journal of Dental and Medical Sciences (IOSR-JDMS)
e-ISSN: 2279 0853, p-ISSN: 2279-0861. Volume 8, Issue 4 (Jul.-Aug. 2013), PP 46-50
www.iosrjournals.org

Quality of life, level of physical activity and depression in dialysis patients
A. Thangamani Ramalingam,[1] Dibeyandu Narayan Bid,[1] Rajiv D. Limbasia,[1] Mandaviya Ushma M,[2]. Jariwala Dimple K,[2]. Patel Dimple M Patel,[2] Vaibhav R.[2]

[1] Faculty members, Sarvajanik College of Physiotherapy, Rampura, Surat
[2] Graduate physiotherapists, Sarvajanik College of Physiotherapy, Surat

www.iosrjournals.org   46 Page
(Title)

Quality of life, level of physical activity and depression in dialysis patients

(Running head)

Common issues:
- A title may be too long, using brackets and abbreviations.
- No novelty and influencing keywords
- May be in question form

2. Abstract
- Abstract should be as short and clear as possible (summary).
- Give a brief introduction or background of the study.
- Explain the exact research questions and the aims of the study
- Give a brief description of the methodology, the results and discussion.
- It may include keywords for index searching of web.
- In other words, the abstract should answer the following questions:
- Why was the study done?
- What is the background of the problem?
- What was done in the study and the findings?
- What conclusions were derived and its implication?

Figure 23.2 describes the structure of the abstract.

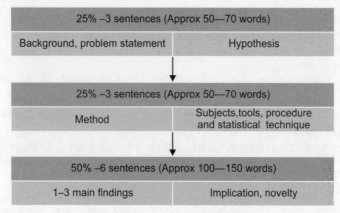

Figure 23.2: Structure of the abstract.

Example:

ABSTRACT

Background: Different current frequencies are considered to produce a different reaction in tissues. But there is still a lack of knowledge about the reactions of tissues on medium frequency electric currents with different frequencies in special groups of diseases or trauma.

Objective: The main objective of the study was to find out the difference of physiological response between normal healthy, chronic low back pain and postoperative pain subjects for a medium frequency (4 KHz) electrical stimuli with 20, 50 and 100 Hz base frequencies.

Method: Readings were taken for sensory, motor and pain threshold with three different frequencies 20 Hz, 50 Hz and 100 Hz for normal healthy, chronic low back pain and postoperative pain subjects. Electrodes were applied over the dorsal and ventral side of the ankle in all the maneuvers. For the normality of the data, Shapiro-Wilk test was done. Statistical analysis was done using IBM SPSS version 20.0 and significance were set at "$p<0.05$".

Result: A multivariate ANOVA test showed significant difference statistically between groups; sensory and the motor threshold for back pain was less than normal and postoperative subjects, irrespective of the frequencies used for stimulation. The post hoc analysis between groups showed that chronic low back pain subjects differ from normal individuals in pain threshold (difference 1.617 mA, $p = .041$).

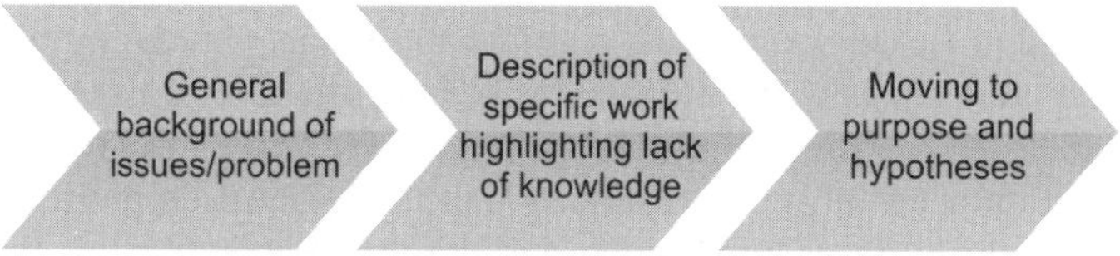

Figure 23.3: Structure of introduction.

> **Conclusion:** The sensory and motor response threshold was more in acute pain subjects and in normal individuals than chronic low back pain subjects. Reduced sensory motor threshold and increased pain threshold in chronic back pain subjects may indicate hyperalgesia and perceptual delay in processing of the electrical stimuli by the nerves system.
>
> **Keywords:** sensory, motor, pain threshold, medium frequency stimuli.

Common issues:
Lack of clarity of results
Results are not supported by statistics
No explanation of the implications
Lack of structure
Irrelevant comments (vague) and self-opinion of author.
References in the abstract.

3. The introduction

It gives some background information, the importance of the study, the rationale behind the research, the limitations of the study and the assumptions of the author with rationale. The introduction part also is important for the researcher to justify the reason behind carrying out the proposed research through evidence gap in the prior knowledge. The structure of introduction is represented schematically (Fig. 23.3).

> **Example:**
> **Introduction**
> Personality plays an important role that effects the academic achievement of college students. A study conducted on undergraduates who completed the Five Factor Inventory Processes and offered their grade point average (GPA) suggested that conscientiousness and agreeableness have a positive relationship with all types of learning styles, whereas neuroticism has an inverse relationship with them all. The Big Five Personality Traits accounted

for 14% of the variance in GPA, suggesting that personality traits make great contributions to academic performance. These results indicate that intellectual curiousness has significant enhancement in academic performance (Komarraju et al, 2011). Study conducted on college students have concluded that hope, which is linked to agreeableness has a positive effect of psychological well being. Individuals high in neurotic tendencies are less likely to display hopeful tendencies and are negatively associated with well-being (Singh, A. K. 2012). Personality can sometimes be flexible and measuring the Big Five Personality Traits for individuals as they enter certain stages of life may predict their educational identity. Recent studies have suggested the likelihood of an individual's personality affecting their educational identity (Klimstra, T. 2012) Academic success as GPA was found to be positively related with Openness to Experience and Conscientiousness and negatively related with Neuroticism. However, no association was identified between traits of emotional intelligence (EI) and GPA. Trait EI also did not make any significant contribution to the predictive ability of the Big Five personality traits (Serdar Tok, et, al. 2008). These findings provide limited evidence for a link between EI and academic performance for this student group. More extensive work on associations between EI, academic success and adjustment throughout medical training would clearly be of interest (Elizabeth J. Austin, et. al. 2005). A study which examined the role of trait emotional intelligence in academic performance and in deviant behavior at school in British secondary education showed that the Trait EI moderated the relationship between cognitive ability and academic performance. In addition, pupils with high trait EI scores were less likely to have had unauthorized absences and less likely to have been excluded from school. Most trait EI effects persisted even after controlling for personality variance. It is concluded that the constellation of emotion-related self-perceived abilities and dispositions that the construct of trait EI encompasses is implicated in academic performance and deviant behavior, with effects that are particularly relevant to vulnerable or disadvantaged adolescents (Petrides KV, et. al. 2004).

The concept of "self-efficacy" is the center of social cognitive theory of a well-known psychologist named Albert Bandura. Bandura's theory emphasizes on the role of observational learning, social experiences and determinism in developing someone's personality.

Self-efficacy is "belief in one's own capabilities to organize and conduct a series of activities required to manage a variety of conditions and situations. According to Bandura, this belief is the determining factor in how to think, feel and behave among the individuals. Bandura discovered that everyone's self-efficacy plays a major role in the way of approaches, views towards the goals, tasks and challenges. Those who have a strong feeling of self-efficacy considered the challenging issues as the problems that ought to be overcome. They feel more commitment to their goals and activities and quickly overcome the senses of despair and frustration. While those who have weaker self-efficacy avoid from doing the challenging works and are focused on the personal frustrations and negative results, and quickly lose their confidence to their own capabilities and abilities (Albert Bandura, 2002). Educating the cognition skills, expressing and controlling the emotions and having the ability to empathy with others; or summarily, emotional intelligence is necessary in school and university periods and in all periods of life for learning in all fields and getting succeed in all aspects of life (Akbarzade, 2004). Moreover there is a positive relationship between self-efficacy feeling and personality traits and responsibility concerning doing homework and high curriculum mean in final exams, job satisfaction and academic achievements in the students (Gion Witorio, et al. 2006))

Significance of the study

The main challenge of educators is to assist students in becoming successful in college. Physiotherapy programs and university officials continue to be very much concerned with the ability of students to successfully complete rigorous and challenging programs. Personality, emotional intelligence play an important role that effects academic achievement and there is minimal research to specifically identify how those traits and factors influence performance of physiotherapy students during their graduation program.

Purpose of the study

The purpose of this study was to improve understanding of the impact of personality traits and emotional intelligence factors on the academic self-efficacy and recent performance of physiotherapy students.

1. To find out the relationship between trait emotional factors and big five personality traits of physiotherapy students.

2. To find out the effect of trait emotional factors and big five personality traits on academic self-efficacy and performance.

Common issues:
Lack of structure
Lack of references or unrelated references
Lack of education and dissemination
Moving directly to specific issues
Missing connection in the order of arranging the knowledge information

4. Literature Review

It is a process of gathering all the information from other sources.

It is a critical and in depth quality evaluation of previous research findings.

Highlights areas of agreement and disagreement.

Example:
Literature review

According to Paraskevi Theofilou 2007, "The study findings indicates that the hemodialysis (HD) patients have poor QoL in their environment and their social relationships than peritoneal dialysis (PD) patients and both groups reported elevated depression. However, HD patients reported more suicidal thoughts and sleep problems compared to PD patients."

According to Maria Carolina Cruz, et. al, 2011, "Quality of life is decreased in renal patients in the early stages of disease. No association was detected between the stages of the disease and the quality of life."

According to Sathvik BS, et. al. 2008, "the QoL of hemodialysis patients is considerably impaired compared to that of the healthy subjects, especially with respect to the physical, psychological and social relationship domains. Renal transplant patients have better QoL in all the four dimensions of the WHOQoL-BREF compared to hemodialysis patients."

According to M, Ginieri-Coccossis, et. al. 2008, "patients in HD treatment modality, particularly those with many years of treatment, were experiencing a more compromised QoL in comparison to PD patients."

Common issues:
Chronological catalog type information of all of the sources
Collection of quotes and paraphrasing from the sources.

5. Methodology

Describes the materials and equipment that used in the research and explain how the data were going to be gathered from the sample.

- Describes randomization techniques in sampling
- Explains the measurement protocol or procedure
- Describe the statistical techniques that were used upon the data.

This section can be written in subgroups like setting, participants, instruments and procedure.

Example:

Methodology

Subjects

Adult male patients aged equal or greater than 18 years with factor viii or ix deficiency and who were willing to participate and willing to give consent from Surat chapter of hemophiliacs were included in the study. Patients with disabilities other than hemophilia were excluded from the study. A nonprobability sampling method was used.

Procedure

The data were collected from the eligible individuals with hemophilia, who gave consent to participate in the study, by getting the self-reported outcome measures filled and the objective functional instrument administered by the researcher.

Outcome measures

WHOBREF Questionnaire: The WHOQOL-BREF consists of 24 facets and provides a profile of scores on four dimensions of quality of life: physical health, psychological, and social relationships, and the environment. WHOQOLBREF is available in both self-administered and interviewer-administered and assisted forms. For patients who did not understand English language were helped with interviewer assisted forms.

Function independence score: The Functional Independence Score in Hemophilia (FISH) was developed as a performance-based assessment tool to objectively measure an individual's functional ability (self-care, transfer and locomotion) for individuals suffering with Hemophilia. It is intended to measure what the person with disability actually does, not what he ought to be able to do, or might be able to do if circumstances were different, or thinks he can do. It can also be used to evaluate change in functional independence over time, or after a therapeutic intervention. The current version of FISH includes the assessment of eight activities: eating, grooming, dressing, chair transfer, squatting, walking, step climbing, and running. Each activity is graded according to the amount of assistance required to perform it.

Statistical analyses

Data collected were cleaned for paucity before the analysis and the categorical variables presented in percentages and numerical variables in terms of mean and standard deviations for the demographical and clinical outcomes. A Pearson correlation analysis was done among QoL, functional independence and joint scores. Significant outcome variables entered in regression analysis to find out the variance after determining the dependent and independent variables theoretically. A mean comparison between mild and moderate bleeding groups was done using non-parametric Mann Whitney U test. A logistic regression analysis was done to find out the significant personal demographical factors for bleeding groups. Data were analyzed using IBM SPSS Statistics for Windows, Version 20.0. Armonk, NY: IBM Corp. Statistical significance was set at $p<0.05$ (Two tailed).

Common issues:

Incomplete statistics

Lack of proper structure or organization of the research process

Inappropriate use of references in place of method description.

6. Results

Presentation of the findings without interpreting or evaluating.

- Include graphs, figures and tables to make the point clear.
- Make a description of exactly what is found and creates a link to the discussion section.

Example:

Tables 3, 4 and 5 show the correlation between the quality of life components, Functional independence measure components and Total joint limitation score of Gilbert joint evaluation of adult hemophiliac individuals. Significantly correlated outcomes were used in regression analysis to find out the proportion of variance between outcomes. Table 6 shows the regression analysis of the significantly related outcomes of QoL, functional independence and Gilbert joint score.

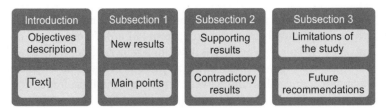

Introduction	Subsection 1	Subsection 2	Subsection 3
Objectives description	New results	Supporting results	Limitations of the study
[Text]	Main points	Contradictory results	Future recommendations

Figure 23.4: Structure of discussion.

Common issues:

Poor and incomplete or too many figures or tables.

Poor presentation of results.

Not fulfilling the criteria of the journal where it is going to be published.

No connection to discussion section.

7. Discussion

It is the interpretation of the research work results.

Comment and criticize the findings and methodology of the research.

Suggest any modifications or improvements of the methodology used and provide recommendations for future researchers.

Authors discuss the results using a personal style. For example, "this study...", "our results...", „we found...", etc.

The structure of the results and discussion (Fig. 23.4).

Example:

Discussion

The current study attempted to find out the difference between sensory, motor and pain threshold among normal, chronic low back pain and acute post- surgical pain subjects. The comparison of the all the three groups showed sensory, the motor threshold for back pain is statistically different from normal individuals and postoperative pain subjects. But pain threshold remained different with normal subjects. All the three thresholds remained same irrespective of the base or beat frequency used for stimulation.

The sequence of the sensory, motor and pain thresholds has been presented by many researchers. The present study results are in support to the result of Lehtela, et. al. that tissues would react differently when stimulated with different frequencies in a different group of subjects characteristic differences of persons with health problems should be confirmed with further testing.[3,4] In one study it was mentioned studies tried to establish the values of sensory, motor and pain of thresholds in the human body and to find out which frequency is good for treatments of a different group of subjects.[13] A likely explanation is that different nerve fiber types have different refractory periods, different periods of hypo- and hyper-excitability, and different recovery times for a medium frequency stimulation.[16,17]

This raises a question that the chronic back pain subjects have hypersensitivity (hyperalgesia). The pain threshold for chronic back pain was little more compared to normal individuals and postoperative pain subjects (no statistical difference). Is it due to perceptual delay due to chronic pain suffering? Or due to peripheral nervous system delay? Moreover, the beat frequencies commonly used in Inferential current treatment may be a cause for over excitation of the nerves tissues respective of the pain condition of the subjects. So it is very important to find out the subgroup of patients with hyperexcitability before applying electrical currents as a treatment modality. As the study used small sample size could be a reason not able to generalize the results. A large sample size study could provide more insight in this context.

Common issues:
The results and observations are not explained in proper manner
Lack of organized structure and poor reference citations
No external implication of the study to the field.

8. Conclusion
It is the final part of your research paper, a personal and positive way of the main findings.
- Gives a brief description of the results and discussion
- Points out the significance of the study and practical uses
- It should not contain bibliographic references.

Example:
Conclusion
The present study shows that the adult hemophiliac patients of Surat chapter reported reasonably good quality of life. The moderate bleed group hemophiliac patients have more of pain and lack of independence. A more concerted, timely and aggressive Physiotherapy principles in the prevention of pain and bleeding for hemophiliac patients and improving their independence may be of more importance and advantage for leading a good quality life.

Common issues:

The author makes general comments and more speculations

Unrelated to the results.

9. References

The citation list must include all of the direct sources referred in the paper.

It helps the researchers to know the work of previous authors in the field.

Citation gives details of authors, title, publishing source and place.

Example:

References

1. Baum, C, Ford W. The wage effects of obesity: a longitudinal study. *Health Econ.* 2004;pp.885-99.
2. Carr D. Friedman M. Is obesity stigmatizing? Body weight, perceived discrimination, and psychological well-being in the United States. *J Health Soc Behav.* 2005;pp.244-59.
3. Dey M, Gmel G, Mohler-Kuo M. Body mass index and health-related quality of life among young Swiss men. *BMC Public Health.* 2013;pp.1-4.
4. Kolotkin R, Crosby R, Kosloski K, Williams G. Development of a Brief Measure to Assess Quality of Life in Obesity. *Obes Res.* 2001;pp.1-3.
5. Kolotkin R, Head S, Brookhart A. Construct validity of the Impact of Weight on Quality of Life questionnaire. *Obes Res.* 1997;5(5), pp.434-41.
6. Le Pen C. et. al. "Specific" scale compared with "generic" scale: a double measurement of the quality of life in a French community sample of obese subjects. *Journal of Epidemiology and Community Health.* 1998;52, pp.445-50.
7. Macardle WD, Katch FI, Katch VL. *EXERCISE PHYSIOLOGY energy, nutrition and human performance.* 4th ed. Wiliam and Wilkins, 2010.
8. Ware J, Kosinsk IM, Keller S. *SF-12* *: How to score the SF-12* * F-12* *F-12* * Physical and Mental Health Summary Scales.* 3rd ed. Lincoln, 1998.
9. WHO. Obesity: Preventing and Managing the Global Epidemic. Geneva, 1998.
10. WHO. Obesity: preventing and managing the global epidemic, 2000.

11. WHO technical Report Series. p.894.
12. WHQOL. The World Health Organization Quality of Life assessment (WHOQOL): Position paper from the World Health Organization, Special Issue on Health-Related Quality of Life: What is it and how should we measure it? *Social Science and Medicine,* 1995.

Common issues:
Incorrectly Formatted References
Failure to Cross-Check References with the body of the article
Poor placement of references.

FURTHER READING

1. Al-Ateeg FA. "Reading medical articles critically. What they do not teach you in medical school." Saudi Med J, 2004;25(4):409-23.
2. Cook DA, et. al. Quality of reporting of experimental studies in medical education: a systematic review. Med Educ, 2007;41(8):737-45.
3. Fahey T, Griffiths S, Peters TJ. Evidence based purchasing: understanding the results of clinical trials and systematic reviews. BMJ 1995; 311:1056–60.
4. Greenhalgh T. "How to read a paper: Assessing the methodological quality of published papers." BMJ, 1997;315(7103):305-08.
5. Loke YK, Derry S. Does anybody read "evidence-based" articles? BMC *Medical Research Methodology,* 2003;3, 14. http://doi.org/10.1186/1471-2288-3-14.
6. Meerpohl JJ, et. al. "[Reporting guidelines are also useful for readers of medical research publications: CONSORT, STARD, STROBE and others]." Dtsch Med Wochenschr, 2009;134(41):2078-83.
7. Subramanyam R. Art of reading a journal article: Methodically and effectively. *Journal of Oral and Maxillofacial Pathology:* JOMFP, 2013;17(1), 65–70. http://doi.org/10.4103/0973-029X.110733.

Methodology in Research Article

METHODOLOGY

Methodology, the etymology of the word refers to 'method' + 'ology'. 'Ology' typically means a discipline of study or a branch of knowledge. Thus technically, 'methodology' is considered to be a study of methods. Methodology and method are not interchangeable. However, there has been a tendency to use methodology as a substitute for the word method. Method is simply a research tool, a component of research – say for example, a qualitative method such as interviews. Methodology is the justification for using a particular research method. A methodology is the design process for carrying out research or the development of a procedure and is not in itself an instrument, or method, or procedure for doing things.

STRATEGY OF METHODOLOGY (TABLE 24.1)

A good methodology should have enough strength to solve the problem of the researcher and contribute to clear results and its interpretation. The materials and methods section is used to describe the design of the study and provide sufficient details so that a competent colleague or researcher can repeat the experiment. A good materials and methods section may enable the readers to evaluate the research performed and replicate the study, if necessary.

Table 24.1: Strategy of methodology

Question	Section of the Article
How the problem is solved by the researcher?	Material and methods
What we found as answers by exploration?	Results
What is the meaning and interpretation of results?	Discussion

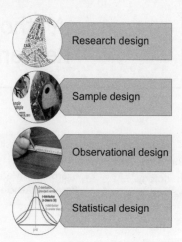

Figure 24.1: Structure of methodology.

STRUCTURE OF METHODOLOGY (FIG. 24.1)

The methodology structure should be strong enough for a research study to get the solution for the hypotheses and objective of the study. It consists of:

1. The research design or type of study required for the problem of interest of the researcher.
2. The sample design or selection, allocation and size of the participants in the study.
3. Observational design or the methods of data collection including observation, interview and measurement.
4. Statistical design or the appropriate mathematical tools to find the results of the collected data.

PURPOSE OF THE METHODOLOGY

The main and important purpose of methodology of a research is to describe the exact procedures that would be carried out to achieve the aim of the project. It further shows a careful and methodical approach to the planned investigation. If a reader reads an article the methodology gives the reader more confidence and provides sufficient detail about the study. It may be more helpful for another researcher to replicate the study precise. Table 24.2 highlights the methodology in a research and corresponding application from the results or purpose. Moreover this improves the validity part of a research as shown in table.

Table 24.2: Purpose of the methodology

Methodology	Purpose of the methodology
Research design	Internal validity
Sampling design	External validity
Observational design	Construct validity
Statistical design	Conclusion validity

PRINCIPLES OF WRITING METHODOLOGY SECTION OF A RESEARCH STUDY

Methodology section is one of the parts of a research and it is a proof that the researcher used scientific method with sufficient validity. The methodology of a research study is expected to answer two main questions which the writer of a research study should mind during the write up. They are:

How was the data collected?

How was the data analyzed?

Writing should be direct and precise.

Normally past tense used for writing.

Include enough information (**data collection equipment and the techniques**) so that others could repeat the experiment and evaluate whether the results are reproducible.

The explanation of the collection and the analysis of data is very important because; readers need to know the reasons why you chose a particular method or procedure instead of others and is valid in the field of study.

Discuss the anticipated problems in the process of the data collection and the steps taken to prevent them.

Present the justification or rationale for the chosen procedures.

The order of the methods section should flow like this:

1. Describing the samples/participants: Present the basic demographic profile of the sample population like age, gender, and the racial composition of the sample.
2. Describing the research design: Type of study, randomization, sampling.
3. Describing the materials used in the study and explaining how the materials and equipment were used for data collection.
4. Protocol: Explaining how you made measurements and what calculations you performed.
5. State which statistical tests were used to analyze the data—Software/Statistical packages used.

EXAMPLES OF METHODOLOGY IN A RESEARCH ARTICLE

1. Difference in sensory, motor and pain threshold for medium frequency electrical stimuli in different pain conditions-A pilot study. Journal of Integrated Health Sciences online ISSN 2347-6494; print–ISSN-2347-6486, Vol IV, Issue II, Dec 2016. www.jihs.com

2. Factors associated with increased body mass index and its impact on health related quality of life of pre obese and obese subjects, Multi-Disciplinary Edu Global Quest (Quarterly), (e-ISSN 2250 – 3048) Volume 5, Issue 2 #18, October 2016 pg 151-165 www.mdegq.com

METHODOLOGY

Subjects

An observational pilot study used non-probability prospective sampling collected data from 20 postoperative pain subjects, 20 normal individuals and 20 chronic low back pain Subjects between the ages of 18 to 65 years who were willing to give consent. Patients who have undergone laparotomy and receiving the postoperative care immediately thereafter; patients who were suffering from low back pain for more than six months duration; and normal healthy individuals without any major illnesses were included in the study. Subjects with any other major illnesses such as trauma, myopathy, neuropathy, epilepsy and diseases which may alter the physiological responses were considered for exclusion.

Tools

Interferential therapy equipment-VECTROSTIM from techno med electronics, Chennai with serial no 341 with medium size rubber electrodes was used to produce medium frequency stimuli with different frequencies.

Procedure

For the present study the subjects were taken from Lockhat Hospital and Sarvajanik College of Physiotherapy, Surat according to our inclusion and exclusion criteria and who gave consent to participate in the study. The study was conducted after the permission and approval from the hospital authority. Readings were taken for sensory, motor and pain threshold using three different amplitude-modulated frequencies (AMF) or base or beat frequencies 20 Hz, 50 Hz and 100 Hz with 4 kHz interferential current (alternating current) for all the three groups. For this, the subjects were asked to lie on a plinth and electrodes were fixed on dorsum and plantar aspect of the foot. Then the intensity of the machine was increased slowly on "1" point basis and the subject was asked to inform the feel of current, the intensity of the machine was noted (sensory threshold) and further when the experimenter perceived the movement of the foot, intensity noted (motor threshold). The current was given further to find out pain threshold when subject self-reported discomfort for a particular intensity (pain threshold). The above said procedure was done for normal healthy individuals and chronic low back pain patients at their first visit; And for postoperative pain cases it was done after 48 hours of surgery.

Data analysis
A multivariate ANOVA was used as primary statistical analysis for Between-group and within-group comparisons. All the analysis was done using IBM SPSS statistics for windows, version 20.0. Armonk, NY: IBM corp. Statistical significance was set at "$p<0.05$"for all statistical analyses.

Methods
Study design
Cross -Sectional study.

Subjects
Data were collected from the residents of Surat who falls under the category of pre-obese and obese undergoing weight reduction training in primary according to the inclusion criteria age: 18-65 years; BMI : >24.9 kg/m.

Tools
Body mass index (BMI)
We calculated BMI from self-reported height and weight and created the following five categories of BMI according to the World Health Organization guidelines underweight (<18.5 kg/m^2), normal weight (18.5–24.9 kg/m^2), preobese (overweight) (25–29.9 kg/m^2), obesity class I/moderate obesity (30–34.9 kg/m^2), and obesity class II/severe obesity (≥ 35 kg/m^2) (WHO 2000), (WHO 1998).

Health-related quality-of-life (HRQoL)
The Short-Form 12 (SF-12) is comprised of 12 items measuring eight concepts: physical functioning, role limitations due to physical health problems, bodily pain, general health, vitality, social functioning,

role limitations due to emotional health, and mental health. These concepts are combined into physical and mental component summary scales that are scored using norm-based methods and transformed so that the general population has a mean of 50 and a standard deviation of 10. (Ware J Jr 1996) (Ware JE 1998)

Physical activity was assessed using the 'International Physical Activity Questionnaire (IPAQ) – short form (low, moderate and high physical activity)

IPAQ comprises a set of 4 questionnaires. Long (5 activity domains asked independently) and short (4 generic items) versions for use by either telephone or self-administered methods are available. The purpose of the questionnaires is to provide common instruments that can be used to obtain internationally comparable data on health–related physical activity.The IPAQ instruments have acceptable measurement properties, at least as good as other established self-reports. Considering the diverse samples in this study, IPAQ has reasonable measurement properties for monitoring population levels of physical activity among 18- to 65-yr-old adults in diverse settings (IPAQ 2005).

Impact of weight on quality of life (IWQOL-Lite) (31-item version)

The IWQOL Lite assesses the impact of weight on quality of life in five areas: Physical Function (11 items), Self-Esteem (7 items), Sexual Life (4 items), Public Distress (5 items), and Work (4 items). (Kolotkin RL 2001) (Kolotkin RL 1995) (Kolotkin RL 1997).

Procedure

The data collection sheet included demographic data and other questionnaires were distributed to 300 Subjects. Consent was taken and objective of the study was explained and instructions were given to fill the questionnaire to the Subjects in prior. Among the 300 only 273 subjects returned the data sheet and 7 were excluded as they were having normal BMI and 266 were considered for data analyses.

Statistical Analyses

Data collected were cleaned for paucity before the analysis and the categorical variables presented in percentages and numerical variables in terms of mean and standard deviations for the demographical and health outcomes. Spearman rank correlation coefficient test was done to explore the magnitude and relationships between HRQoL, BMI, and physical activity level and socio-demographic characteristics.

A Logistic regression analysis was done to find out the significant personal demographical factors for obese subjects. To evaluate the difference of Impact of weight on QoL between pre-obese and obese subjects an independent sample t test was done. Data were analyzed using IBM SPSS Statistics for Windows, Version 20.0. Armonk, NY: IBM Corp. Statistical significance was set at $p < 0.05$ (Two tailed).

FURTHER READING

1. DeMaria AN. How do I get a paper accepted? J Am Coll Cardiol. 2007;17:1666–7.
2. Kallet RH. How to write the methods section of a research paper. Respiratory Care 2004;49(10):1229-1232.
3. Lundberg GD. How to write a medical paper to get it published in a good journal. Med Gen Med. 2005;4:36.
4. Ng KH, Peh WC. Writing the materials and methods." Singapore Med J 2008;49(11):856-858.
5. Ohwovoriole AE. Writing biomedical manuscripts part I: fundamentals and general rules. West Afr J Med 2011;30(3):151-157.
6. Setiati S, Harimurti K. Writing for scientific medical manuscript: a guide for preparing manuscript submitted to biomedical journals. Acta Med Indones 2007;39(1):50-55.
7. Zeiger M. Essentials of writing biomedical research papers. New York: McGraw-Hill; 1991;113–138.

Critical Appraisal Tools

CRITICAL APPRAISAL

Critical appraisal is the process of careful and systematic assessment of the outcome of scientific research (evidence) to judge its trustworthiness, value and relevance in a particular context. Evidence that is of trustworthy value would help in effective solution to a problem. Critical appraisal looks at the way a study is conducted and examines factors such as internal validity, generalizability and relevance. It aims to bring out the evidence generated from research to be of value to make a decision for a problem.

For the on-going release of research reports in any area of scientific evaluation, Critical appraisal is the use of explicit, transparent methods to assess the data in published research, applying the rules of evidence to factors such as internal validity, adherence to reporting standards, conclusions and generalizability. Thus critical appraisal methods form a central part of the systematic review process by synthesizing effective evidence and process of keeping update with the knowledge. It can be said that it is an on-going process of scientific evaluation. They are used in evidence-based healthcare training to assist clinical decision-making, and are increasingly used in evidence-based social care and education provision.

PURPOSE OF CRITICAL APPRAISAL

Critical appraisal is the systematic evaluation of clinical research papers in order to establish answers for the following questions:
• Does this study address a clearly focused question/hypothesis?

- Did the study use valid methods to address this question/methodo-logy?
- Are the valid results of this study important/external validity?
- Are these valid, important results applicable to my patient or popu-lation/clinical application/generalization of results to population?
- If the answer to any of these questions is "no", you can save yourself the trouble of reading the rest of it.

GENERAL APPRAISAL QUESTIONS

In practical terms from the above mentioned questions, when a physiotherapy practitioner intends to appraise a research article he must be interested to get the answers for the following questions:

1. How was the outcome measured?
2. Is that a reliable way to measure?
3. How large was the effect size?
4. What implications does the study have for your practice? Is it relevant?
5. Can the results be applied to your clinical question or organization?

CHECKLISTS FOR SPECIFIC STUDY DESIGNS

The clinician can consider using the following appraisal questionnaires/ checklists for specific study designs:

- Appraisal of a meta-analysis or systematic review
- Appraisal of a controlled study
- Appraisal of a cohort or panel study
- Appraisal of a case control study
- Appraisal of a cross-sectional study (survey)
- Appraisal of a qualitative study
- Appraisal of a case study
- Checklist for analytical cross-sectional studies
- Checklist for quasi-experimental studies (non-randomized experi-mental studies)
- Checklist for prevalence studies.

1. An example: A critical appraisal checklist for an article on treat-ment or prevention.

Study Design: Randomized Controlled Trial

Adapted from: Critical Appraisal Skills Programme (CASP), Public Health Resource Unit, Institute of Health Science, Oxford.

The reader or the appraiser should get the response for the following items on the below format:

	Yes		Can't tell		No

DOES THIS STUDY ADDRESS A CLEAR QUESTION?
1. Were the following clearly stated:
- Patients
- Intervention
- Comparison Intervention
- Outcome(s).

ARE THE RESULTS OF THIS SINGLE TRIAL VALID?
A. The main questions to answer:
2. Was the assignment of patients to treatments randomized?
3. Was the randomization list concealed? Can you tell?
4. Were all subjects who entered the trial accounted for at it's conclusion?
5. Were they analyzed in the groups to which they were randomized, i.e. intention-to-treat analysis.

B. Some finer points to address:
6. Were subjects and clinicians 'blind' to which treatment was being received, i.e. could they tell?
7. Aside from the experimental treatment, were the groups treated equally?
8. Were the groups similar at the start of the trial?

WHAT WERE THE RESULTS?

	Outcome event		Total
	Yes	No	
Experimental group	a	b	a + b
Control group	c	d	c + d

Experimental event rate = risk of outcome event in experimental group = EER = $a/(a + b)$ Control event rate = risk of outcome event in control group = CER = $c/(c + d)$

Relative risk (RR) = EER/CER

Odds ratio (OR) = ad/bc

Relative risk reduction (RRR) = (CER - EER)/CER or 1 - RR

Absolute risk reduction (ARR) = CER - EER

Number needed to treat (NNT) = 1/ARR = 1/(CER - EER)

9. How large was the treatment effect? Consider: How were the results expressed (RRR, NNT, etc.).
10. How precise were the results? Were the results presented with confidence intervals?

CAN I APPLY THESE VALID, IMPORTANT RESULTS TO MY PATIENT?

11. Do these results apply to my patient? · Is my patient so different from those in the trial that the results don't apply?
    How great would the benefit of therapy be for my particular patient?
12. Are my patient's values and preferences satisfied by the intervention offered?
    Do I have a clear assessment of my patient's values and preferences?
    Are they met by this regimen and its potential consequences?

TERMINOLOGIES USED FOR CRITICAL APPRAISAL

Randomized controlled trial (RCT): Clinical trial where at least two treatment groups are compared. One must be a control group, e.g. receiving standard care or a placebo treatment. Allocation to a group must be random and unbiased.

Randomization: Process of allocating individuals to the alternative treatments in a clinical trial, avoiding bias. This should produce groups which are similar, except for the treatment of interest.

Blinding: The process of ensuring that participants or researchers (single-blind) or participants and researchers (double-blind) are unaware of which treatment group participants have been randomized to, reducing the possibility of bias in the results.

Intention-to-treat analysis (ITT): All patients allocated to one arm of a RCT are analyzed in that arm, whether or not they completed the prescribed treatment/regimen.

Quantifying the Risk of Benefit/Harm in RCTs

Experimental event rate (EER): Risk (or chance) of outcome event in experimental group.

Control event rate (CER): Risk (or chance) of outcome event in control group.

Relative risk (RR): A measure of the chance of the event occurring in the experimental group relative to it occurring in the control group.

Relative risk reduction (RRR): The difference in the proportion of events between the control and experimental groups, relative to the proportion of events in the control group. It can also be calculated as 1-RR.

Absolute risk reduction (ARR): The absolute difference between the risk of the event in the control and experimental groups.

Number needed to treat (NNT): The number of patients who needed to be treated to prevent the occurrence of one adverse event (e.g. complication, death) or promote the occurrence of one beneficial event (e.g. cessation of smoking).

Ideal NNT=1; The higher the NNT, the less effective the treatment

Confidence interval: For whatever effect being measures (e.g. RR, RRR, ARR, NTT) the confidence interval is the range of values within which the "true" value in the population is found. Generally expressed as a 95% confidence interval, i.e. If the same trial repeated hundreds of times would not yield the same results every time. But on average the results would be within a certain range. A 95% confidence interval means that there is a 95% chance that the true size of effect will lie within this range.

Odds of outcome: In each patient group, the number of patients with an outcome divided by the number of patients without the outcome.

Odds ratio: Odds of outcome in treatment group divided by odds of outcome in control group.

If the outcome is negative, an effective treatment will have an odds ratio <1;
If the outcome is positive, an effective treatment will have an odds ratio >1.

(In case control studies, the odds ratio refers to the odds in favor of exposure to a particular factor in cases divided by the odds in favor of exposure in controls).

2. **An example**: STROBE Statement—Checklist of items that should be included in reports of *cross-sectional studies.*

1. **Title and abstract**
    a. Indicate the study's design with a commonly used term in the title or the abstract.
    b. Provide in the abstract an informative and balanced summary of what was done and what was found.

Introduction

2. Background/rationale: Explain the scientific background and rationale for the investigation being reported.
3. Objectives: State specific objectives, including any prespecified hypotheses.

Methods

4. Study design: Present key elements of study design early in the paper.
5. Setting: Describe the setting, locations, and relevant dates, including periods of recruitment, exposure, follow-up, and data collection.
6. Participants: Give the eligibility criteria, and the sources and methods of selection of participants.
7. Variables: Clearly define all outcomes, exposures, predictors, potential confounders, and effect modifiers. Give diagnostic criteria, if applicable.
8*. Data sources/measurement: For each variable of interest, give sources of data and details of methods of assessment (measurement). Describe comparability of assessment methods if there is more than one group.
9. Bias: Describe any efforts to address potential sources of bias.
10. Study size: Explain how the study size was arrived at.
11. Quantitative variables: Explain how quantitative variables were handled in the analyses. If applicable, describe which groupings were chosen and why.
12. Statistical methods:
    a. Describe all statistical methods, including those used to control for confounding.
    b. Describe any method used to examine subgroups and interactions.
    c. Explain how missing data were addressed.
    d. If applicable, describe analytical methods taking account of sampling strategy.
    e. Describe any sensitivity analyses.

Results

13*. Participants:
    a. Report numbers of individuals at each stage of study—e.g. numbers potentially eligible, examined for eligibility, confirmed

*Give information separately for exposed and unexposed groups.

eligible, included in the study, completing follow-up, and
analyzed.

  b. Give reasons for non-participation at each stage.

  c. Consider use of a flow diagram.

14*. Descriptive data

  a. Give characteristics of study participants (e.g. demographic,
  clinical, social) and information on exposures and potential
  confounders.

  b. Indicate number of participants with missing data for each
  variable of interest.

15*. Outcome data: Report numbers of outcome events or summary
measures.

16. Main results:

  a. Give unadjusted estimates and, if applicable, confounder-
  adjusted estimates and their precision (e.g. 95% confidence
  interval). Make clear which confounders were adjusted for and
  why they were included.

  b. Report category boundaries when continuous variables were
  categorized.

  c. If relevant, consider translating estimates of relative risk into
  absolute risk for a meaningful time period.

17. Other analyses: Report other analyses done—e.g. analyses of
subgroups and interactions, and sensitivity analyses.

Discussion

18. Key results: Summarise key results with reference to study
objectives.

19. Limitations: Discuss limitations of the study, taking into account
sources of potential bias or imprecision. Discuss both direction
and magnitude of any potential bias.

20. Interpretation: Give a cautious overall interpretation of results
considering objectives, limitations, multiplicity of analyses,
results from similar studies, and other relevant evidence.

21. Generalisability: Discuss the generalisability (external validity)
of the study results.

Other information

22. Funding: Give the source of funding and the role of the funders
for the present study and, if applicable, for the original study on
which the present article is based.

*Give information separately for exposed and unexposed groups.

FEW TOOLS/SITES FOR CRITICAL APPRAISAL (TABLE 25.1)

Table 25.1: Critical appraisal tools

Study type	Tools
For **Randomized Controlled Trials**	AGREE - http://www.agreecollaboration.org/.
	Alberta University Evidence Based Medicine Toolkit - http://www.ebm.med.ualberta.ca/
	CASP - http://www.sph.nhs.uk/what-we-do/public-health-workforce/resources/critical-appraisals-skills-programme.
	PEDro scalehttp://www.pedro.org.au/english/downloads/pedro-scale/
	The CONSORT statement- http://www.consort-statement.org/consort-statement/
	The JADAD score http://onlinelibrary.wiley.com/doi/10.1002/9780470988343.app1/pdf
	CATwalk - http://www.library.ualberta.ca/subject/healthsciences/catwalk/index.cfm
	CEBMH - http://cebmh.warne.ox.ac.uk/cebmh/education_critical_appraisal.htm
	Centre for Evidence Based Medicine - http://www.cebm.net
	CLIST Resources for Critical Appraisal - http://www.londonlinks.nhs.uk/groups/clinical-librarians-informationskills-trainers-group/trainers-toolkit/resources-for-critical-appraisal
	Scottish Intercollegiate Guidelines Network (SIGN): • http://www.sign.ac.uk/
	AMSTAR - https://amstar.ca/Amstar_Checklist.php
	Shea BJ, Reeves BC, Wells G, Thuku M, Hamel C, Moran J, Moher D, Tugwell P, Welch V, Kristjansson E, Henry DA. AMSTAR 2: a critical appraisal tool for systematic reviews that include randomised or non-randomised studies of healthcare interventions, or both. BMJ. 2017 Sep 21;358:j4008.
For **Non-Randomized Controlled Trials**	TheTRENDstatement- http://www.cdc.gov/trendstatement/docs/AJPH_Mar2004_Trendstatement.pdf
	McMaster Critical Review Form - Quantitative Studies- http://www.unisa.edu.au/Global/Health/Sansom/Documents/iCAHE/CATs/McMasters_Quantitative%20review.pdf

Contd...

Contd...

Study type	Tools
For **Other Quantitative Research**	CASP- http://www.casp-uk.net/#!casp-tools-checklists/c18f8
	Evaluation Tool for Quantitative Research Studies- http://usir.salford.ac.uk/12969/
	GATE - https://www.fmhs.auckland.ac.nz/en/soph/about/our-departments/epidemiology-and-biostatistics/research/epiq/evidence-based-practice-and-cats.html
	The STARD Checklist- http://www.stard-statement.org/
	READER Critical Appraisal Tool- http://www.ncbi.nlm.nih.gov/pmc/articles/PMC1238789/pdf/brjgenprac00035-0039.pdf
	ReLIANT - http://eprints.rclis.org/8082/
	STROBE Statement- http://www.strobe-statement.org/index.php?id=strobe-home
For **case studies**	CASP -http://www.casp-uk.net/#!casp-tools-checklists/c18f8
	MINORS Tool- http://cobe.paginas.ufsc.br/files/2014/10/MINORS.pdf
	The Single-Case Experimental Design (SCED) Scale - http://www.psycbite.com/docs/The_SCED_Scale.pdf
For **Systematic Reviews**	CASP -http://www.casp-uk.net/#!casp-tools-checklists/c18f8
	AMSTAR- -http://www.ncbi.nlm.nih.gov/pmc/articles/PMC1810543/pdf/1471-2288-7-10.pdf.
	Systematic Review (of Therapy) Worksheet - http://ktclearinghouse.ca/cebm/teaching/worksheets/sr
	ARIF Checklist-

FURTHER READING

1. Bialocerkowski AE, Grimmer KA, Milanese SF, Kumar VS. Application of current research evidence to clinical physiotherapy practice. Journal of Allied Health. 2004;33(4):230-7.
2. Crowe M, Sheppard L. A review of critical appraisal tools show they lack rigor: Alternative tool structure is proposed. J Clin Epidemiol 2011;64(1):79-89.
3. Grimmer KA, Milanese S, Bialocerkowski AE, Kumar S. Producing and implementing evidence in clinical practice: the therapies' dilemma. Physiotherapy. 2004.

4. Katrak P, Bialocerkowski AE, Massy-Westropp N, Kumar VS, Grimmer KA. A systematic review of the content of critical appraisal tools. *BMC Medical Research Methodology,* 2004;4, 22. http://doi.org/10.1186/1471-2288-4-22.
5. Moseley AM, Herbert RD, Sherrington C, Maher CG. Evidence for physiotherapy practice: A survey of the Physiotherapy Evidence Database. Physiotherapy Evidence Database (PEDro) Australian Journal of Physiotherapy. 2002;48:43–50.
6. National Health and Medical Research Council How to Use the Evidence: Assessment and Application of Scientific Evidence Canberra. 2000.

Critical Appraisal of Clinical Trials

CRITICAL APPRAISAL

"Critical appraisal, an important element of evidence-based practice, is the process of carefully and systematically examining research to judge its trustworthiness, and its value and relevance in a particular context." — *(Burls 2009)*

It is very important for a practicing physiotherapist to know whether the research study or clinical trial results are clinically relevant or just an unjustified scientific claim.

TYPES OF TRIALS

A clinical trial otherwise also called as randomized controlled trial (RCT) is a gold standard in testing the efficacy of an intervention in which participants are either randomly or non-randomly allocated to a test treatment and a control. Information from RCT is considered high in the level of evidence table in that the probability of accepting or rejecting the research hypothesis is purely left to a process of chance, and hence the reliability of the result. Moreover the randomized trial involves concurrent enrolment and follow-up of both groups. Based on randomization process there are two types of clinical trials.

1. Randomized clinical trials (RCTs): Allocation to the different treatment groups of a trial is done through proper randomization process.
2. Non-randomized clinical trials: Allocation to the different treatment groups of a trial is not done through proper randomization process.

RANDOMIZED CLINICAL TRIAL (RCT) DESIGNS

As seen before in the chapter on research designs, based on the way the treatment or intervention are altered within the groups, in randomized designs, classification are done into as follows:

1. Factorial design: Factorial study designs are used where two or more treatment factors are being compared simultaneously and only relative comparisons can be made between the groups involved.

2. Cross-over design: Treatment given to groups are 'switched' after a specified period.

3. Cluster random design: In this design actual treatment centers and not individual subjects are randomized to the respective allocated treatments. All the subjects in a center therefore receive the same treatment to which that center was allocated.

4. n-of-1 trials-competing treatments are randomized to different time periods for each trial subject. Each subject is then administered the respective treatments including the placebo treatment sequentially over allocated time periods.

5. Open trials: In this kind of trials sample size formula, that is, significance level, required power and a would-be acceptable effect size, are defined before the start of the trial. As subjects are then recruited into the trial, accumulated data are inspected continually or periodically until the pre-specified trial end-point conditions are met.

Nevertheless, inference from any type of randomized study trial would be useful in making reliable decision in a clinical scenario. At any point of time, for most of the randomized researches, a specific type of randomized study design is chosen from the above mentioned five designs, depending upon the question asked by the researcher. Hence it was also decided by the authors to keep this current chapter separately on critical appraisal of RCTs given the importance of RCTs in EBP. Hence a tool or checklist looking for all the possible effects in an RCT is deemed to be an effective tool.

METHODS OF RANDOMIZATION

Various types of randomization methods are used depending on the need of the research and as deemed appropriate by the researcher for the specific design. Broadly, fixed and adaptive randomizations are the two major methods used.

1. **Fixed Randomization Methods:** Simple randomization-tossing coin, random number tables or computer generated random numbers.

   Block randomization-permuted blocks are used in a random order and deliberately in different length, e.g. ABAB- ABBBA-BAAB.

   Stratified randomization: To ensure a balance of the stratification factors, e.g. gender groups, age based groups.

   Randomized consent method: To verify the effects of informed consent on treatment efficacy this method is used.

2. **Adaptive Randomization Methods:** The probability of allocated to any group is not fixed throughout the process.

   Play the winner-first subject is allocated by a simple randomization procedure and thereafter; every subsequent allocation is based on the success or failure of the immediate predecessor subject.

   Minimization: It involves identifying a few important prognostic factors in a trial and then applying a weighting system to them. Minimization becomes impractical when more than 3–4 prognostic factors are involved

NON-RANDOMIZATION PROCEDURES

The following are commonly used for randomization of subjects in research by the researchers. But methodology or procedure used is considered not to be true randomization as the allocation process is prone for observer bias for an external observer in the research group.

- Alternate allocation
- Geographical distribution
- Cluster allocation
- Odd/even number allocation
- Based on date of birth/surnames/alphabetical orders.

STRENGTH AND WEAKNESS/ISSUES OF RCT DESIGNS

The critical appraisal of an RCT should provide answers to the following queries like whether the study design used is methodologically sound enough to be considered as RCT? What do the results convey to the reader and whether the results are useful for a practicing therapist? The therapist should need to look primarily on biases and methodology to identify the strength of an RCT. The important points to be noted for critical appraisal of an RCT are given below along with reasoning and solutions:

Sample Size Calculation Stated in the Study

A trial should be big enough with appropriate sample size to have a high chance of detecting a worthwhile effect if it exists for the proposed hypothesis.

Selection Bias

Systematic differences between baseline characteristics of the groups.

Solution: Random sequence generation.

Concealed allocation (Patients and investigators enrolling the patients shouldn't know which group the next patient is going to; can't know the sequence).

Selection methods: Randomization in allocation–this would handle the issue of confounding factors of the study.

[Acceptable methods of randomization include random numbers, either from tables or computer generated [Schulz KF, Grimes DA. Blinding in randomised trials: hiding who got what. Lancet (London, England). 2002;359(9307):696-700]. Unacceptable methods include last digit of date of birth, date seen in clinic, etc. [Stewart LA, Parmar MK. Bias in the analysis and reporting of randomized controlled trials. International Journal of Technology Assessment in Health Care. 1996;12(2):264-75].

Homogenous groups are compared: No distribution bias.

Baseline characteristics: Both the control and the intervention group should be broadly similar in factors like age, sex distribution and level of illness.

Inclusion and Exclusion Bias

Systematic difference in selection process.

Solution: Proper inclusion and exclusion criteria.

Detection Bias

Systematic differences in how are outcomes assessed? The same way for both groups.

Solution: blinded outcome assessments. The investigator measuring outcome should not know about the groups in the study.

Performance Bias

Systematic differences in how patients are treated and in how patients behave during a study other than the intervention- Groups treated equally apart from the treatments.

Solution: Blinding.
Blinding: Reduces the bias of experimenter observation.
Blinding means masking who is getting treatment and control.
Single blinding: Participants do not know.
Double blinding: Neither the participants nor those giving the intervention know.
Triple blinding: Statisticians doing the analysis also do not know.

Standardized Procedures followed in Administering the Treatment Protocols

Reliability and validity of outcome measures used.
Are the outcomes explicitly described? (Primary and secondary outcome measures).
Are all clinically relevant outcomes reported?
Duration of the study: Adequate follow up logically needed to find a difference.

Attrition Bias

Systematic differences in withdrawals from the study.
Solution: Minimal loss to follow-up; an intention-to-treat analysis conducted.

Less than 5%—little bias
5 to 20%—small bias
More than 20%—serious threats to validity.

[Intention to treat analysis: All data of participants including those who withdraw from the trial should be analyzed. Failure to do so may lead to underestimation/overestimation of results (Hollis and Campbell 1999)].

Dropouts management methods
- Worst case scenario method: The researcher assumes a poor outcome for dropouts in fared better group and good outcome for fared worse group.
- Last data carried forward method: The last recorded data are carried forward to the end of trial.

Appropriate Statistical Tests

Whether the statistical tests are relevant and described the effect, and assessed significance effectively.

Information Bias

Surrogate end points: Using accessory or irrelevant outcome measures in place of actual outcomes to support the hypothesis.

Solution: clinically meaningful outcomes should be used.

[E.g. In knee rehabilitation we should show improvement in functions like gait, posture, balance, etc., not only by a change in range of motion score difference.]

Hawthorne Effect

The effect felt by the subjects because of the presence of the experimenter or the therapist who delivers treatment. In general subjects show positive responses to treatment to satisfy the therapist irrespective of absence of real change. It is also due to the result of being in an experimental trial and feeling good for that. This effect may influence both experimental and control groups.

Solution: A third silent group can be used for comparison.

Interim Analyses

To confirm when to stop recruiting subjects for the study or to verify whether the calculated sample size before the study is having enough power to generalize the results or we need more sample size.

Solution: smaller p value significance in the earlier interim analyses may be more useful for the researcher to decide the sample size.

Reporting Bias

Selective reporting of the results or not reporting some results purposefully to enhance the hypothesis what a researcher intended to prove in the study.

Different Biases in RCTs (Greenhalgh 2001)

Figure 26.1 lists the possible biases in an RCT.

ESSENTIAL STATISTICS FOR APPRAISAL OF CLINICAL TRIALS (TABLE 26.1)

It is very important for a researcher to quantify the risk of benefit/harm in RCTs so that the results can be easily generalized and used for the right clinical purpose. The appropriate type of test statistic presented will depend on what type of outcome was measured. For dichotomous outcomes, the results can be expressed in many ways. The following calculations are of more value in this regard.

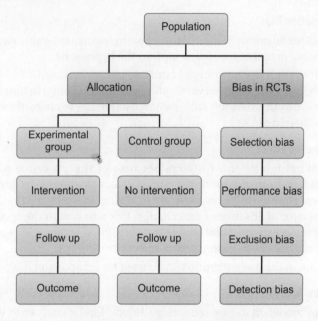

Figure 26.1: Different biases in RCTs.

Table 26.1: Essential statistics

Relative risk (RR) — risk of the outcome in the treatment group/risk of the outcome in the control group	**Absolute risk increase (ARI)** — risk of the outcome in the treatment group-risk of the outcome in the control group
Absolute risk reduction (ARR) — risk of the outcome in the control group – risk of the outcome in the treatment group.	**Number needed to treat (NNT)** — inverse of the ARR and is calculated as 1/ARR
Relative risk reduction — absolute risk reduction/risk of the outcome in the control group.	**Number needed to harm (NNH)** — inverse of the ARI and is calculated as 1/ARI Risk-benefit analysis
Relative risk increase — absolute risk increase/risk of the outcome in the control group.	

CRITICAL APPRAISAL TOOL OF AN RCT STUDY

The readers are advised to apply the scale to RCTs done in various physiotherapy disciplines to make themselves develop the skill of critical appraisal. The PEDro scale was developed by the creators of PEDro (The Physiotherapy Evidence Database).

Last amended June 21st, 1999.

PEDro Scale (Table 26.2)

The PEDro scale is based on the Delphi list developed by Verhagen and colleagues at the Department of Epidemiology, University of Maastricht (Verhagen AP, et al, (1998). The Delphi list: a criteria list for quality assessment of randomized clinical trials for conducting systematic reviews developed by Delphi consensus. Journal of Clinical Epidemiology, 51(12):1235–41.

The complete description of PEDro scale is presented here the way it is given in their website source. The readers can refer the site directly for more details:

"The purpose of the PEDro scale is to help the users of the PEDro database rapidly identify which of the known or suspected randomized clinical trials (RCTs or CCTs) archived on the PEDro database are likely to be internally valid (criteria 2–9), and could have sufficient statistical information to make their results interpretable (criteria 10–11). An additional criterion (criterion 1) that relates to the external validity

Table 26.2: PEDro scale

1. Eligibility criteria were specified	no ❑ yes ❑ where:
2. Subjects were randomly allocated to groups, (in a crossover study, subjects were randomly allocated an order in which treatments were received)	no ❑ yes ❑ where:
3. Allocation was concealed	no ❑ yes ❑ where:
4. The groups were similar at baseline regarding the most important prognostic indicators	no ❑ yes ❑ where:
5. There was blinding of all subjects	no ❑ yes ❑ where:
6. There was blinding of all therapists who administered the therapy	no ❑ yes ❑ where:
7. There was blinding of all assessors who measured at least one key outcome	no ❑ yes ❑ where:
8. Measures of at least one key outcome were obtained from more than 85% of the subjects initially allocated to groups	no ❑ yes ❑ where:
9. All subjects for whom outcome measures were available received the treatment or control condition as allocated or, where this was not the case, data for at least one key outcome was analysed by "intention to treat"	no ❑ yes ❑ where:
10. The results of between-group statistical comparisons are reported for at least one key outcome	no ❑ yes ❑ where:
11. The study provides both point measures and measures of variability for at least one key outcome	no ❑ yes ❑ where:

(or "generalisability" or "applicability" of the trial) has been retained so that the Delphi list is complete, but this criterion will not be used to calculate the PEDro score reported on the PEDro website.

The PEDro scale should not be used as a measure of the "validity" of a study's conclusions. In particular, we caution users of the PEDro scale that studies which show significant treatment effects and which score highly on the PEDro scale do not necessarily provide evidence that the treatment is clinically useful. Additional considerations include whether the treatment effect was big enough to be clinically worthwhile, whether the positive effects of the treatment outweigh its negative effects, and the cost-effectiveness of the treatment. The scale should not be used to compare the "quality" of trials performed in different areas of therapy, primarily because it is not possible to satisfy all scale items in some areas of physiotherapy practice. Notes on administration of the PEDro scale: All criteria Points are only awarded when a criterion is clearly satisfied. If on a literal reading of the trial report it is possible that a criterion was not satisfied, a point should not be awarded for that criterion.

Criterion for Administration of PEDro Scale

Criterion 1 This criterion is satisfied if the report describes the source of subjects and a list of criteria used to determine who was eligible to participate in the study.

Criterion 2 A study is considered to have used random allocation if the report states that allocation was random. The precise method of randomization need not be specified. Procedures such as coin-tossing and dice-rolling should be considered random. Quasi-randomization allocation procedures such as allocation by hospital record number or birth date, or alternation, do not satisfy this criterion.

Criterion 3 Concealed allocations means that the person who determined if a subject was eligible for inclusion in the trial was unaware, when this decision was made, of which group the subject would be allocated to. A point is awarded for this criteria, even if it is not stated that allocation was concealed, when the report states that allocation was by sealed opaque envelopes or that allocation involved contacting the holder of the allocation schedule who was "off-site".

Criterion 4 At a minimum, in studies of therapeutic interventions, the report must describe at least one measure of the severity of the condition being treated and at least one (different) key outcome measure at baseline. The rater must be satisfied that the groups' outcomes would not be expected to differ, on the basis of baseline differences in prognostic variables alone, by a clinically significant amount. This criterion is satisfied even if only baseline data of study completers are presented.

Criteria 4, 7–11 Key outcomes are those outcomes which provide the primary measure of the effectiveness (or lack of effectiveness) of the therapy. In most studies, more than one variable is used as an outcome measure.

Criterion 5–7 Blinding means the person in question (subject, therapist or assessor) did not know which group the subject had been allocated to. In addition, subjects and therapists are only considered to be "blind" if it could be expected that they would have been unable to distinguish between the treatments applied to different groups. In trials in which key outcomes are self-reported (e.g. visual analogue scale, pain diary), the assessor is considered to be blind if the subject was blind.

Criterion 8 This criterion is only satisfied if the report explicitly states both the number of subjects initially allocated to groups and the number of subjects from whom key outcome measures were obtained. In trials in which outcomes are measured at several points in time, a key outcome must have been measured in more than 85% of subjects at one of those points in time.

Criterion 9 An intention to treat analysis means that, where subjects did not receive treatment (or the control condition) as allocated, and where measures of outcomes were available, the analysis was performed as if subjects received the treatment (or control condition) they were allocated to. This criterion is satisfied, even if there is no mention of analysis by intention to treat, if the report explicitly states that all subjects received treatment or control conditions as allocated.

Criterion 10 A between-group statistical comparison involves statistical comparison of one group with another. Depending on the design of the study, this may involve comparison of two or more treatments, or comparison of treatment with a control condition. The analysis may be a simple comparison of outcomes measured after the treatment was administered, or a comparison of the change in one group with the change in another (when a factorial analysis of variance has been used to analyze the data, the latter is often reported as a group × time interaction). The comparison may be in the form hypothesis testing (which provides a "p" value, describing the probability that the groups differed only by chance) or in the form of an estimate (for example, the mean or median difference, or a difference in proportions, or number needed to treat, or a relative risk or hazard ratio) and its confidence interval.

Criterion 11 A point measure is a measure of the size of the treatment effect. The treatment effect may be described as a difference in group outcomes, or as the outcome in (each of) all groups. Measures of variability include standard deviations, standard errors, confidence intervals, interquartile ranges (or other quartile ranges), and ranges. Point measures and/or measures of variability may be provided graphically (e.g. SDs may be given as error bars in a Figure) as long as it is clear what is being graphed (e.g. as long as it is clear whether error bars represent SDs or SEs). Where outcomes are categorical, this criterion is considered to have been met if the number of subjects in each category is given for each group".

FURTHER READING

1. Higgins JPT, et. al. The Cochrane Collaboration's tool for assessing risk of bias in randomised trials. BMJ 2011;343.
2. Jüni P, Altman DG, Egger M. Systematic reviews in health care: assessing the quality of controlled clinical trials. BMJ 2001;323:42-6.
3. Maher CG, Sherrington C, Herbert RD, et al. Reliability of the PEDro scale for rating quality of randomized controlled trials. Phys Ther. 2003;83:713-21.
4. Moher D, Jadad AR, Nichol G, Penman M, Tugwell P, Walsh S. Assessing the quality of randomized controlled trials—an annotated bibliography of scales and checklists. Controlled Clin Trials 1995;12:62-73.
5. Susan Armijo Olivo, Luciana Gazzi Macedo, Inae Caroline Gadotti, Jorge Fuentes, Tasha Stanton, David J Magee. Scales to Assess the Quality of Randomized Controlled Trials: A Systematic Review. Physical Therapy, Volume 88, Issue 2: 2008; 156–75, https://doi.org/10.2522/ptj.20070147.
6. Verhagen AP, de Vet HC, de Bie RA, et. al. The art of quality assessment of RCTs included in systematic reviews. J Clin Epidemiol. 2001;54:651-54.

Systematic Review and Meta-analysis

INTRODUCTION TO SYSTEMATIC REVIEW

A systematic review is a scientific tool that can be used to appraise, summarise, and communicate the results and implications of otherwise unmanageable quantities of research. As a scientific tool it can be applied on any type of literature – epidemiological studies, RCTs, observational studies, diagnostic tests etc., and it is a description of the author's step by step findings on the literature related to the topic of interest or question. To this end, systematic reviews may or may not include a statistical synthesis called meta-analysis, depending on whether the studies are similar enough so that combining their results is meaningful. As systematic reviews attempt to consider all studies published on a given clinical question, conclusions are drawn based on all the available evidence, and a thorough overview of the body of knowledge can be presented. As a textbook designed for therapeutics, most of the information in this chapter relates to the intervention review. However, where required, review information for other design studies are mentioned in the chapter.

Definitions

- According to Straus, et al (2005), "A systematic review is a summary of the medical literature that uses explicit methods to systematically search, critically appraise and synthesize the world literature on a specific issue."
- "Systematic review - identifies and critically appraises all research on a specific topic, and combines valid studies; increasingly important in evidence based medicine; different from review article

(which is a summary of more than one paper on a specific topic, and which may or may not be comprehensive). Meta-analysis - a systematic review that uses quantitative methods to summarise the results." — (Bandolier 2004; NCBI 2010)

- "A review of a clearly formulated question that uses systematic and explicit methods to identify, select, and critically appraise relevant research, and to collect and analyse data from the studies that are included in the review. Statistical methods (meta-analysis) may or may not be used to analyse and summarise the results of the included studies." — (Cochrane Collaboration, 2014)

PRISMA-P (Preferred Reporting Items for Systematic review and Meta-analysis Protocols) Definitions

Systematic review

"A systematic review attempts to collate all relevant evidences that fits pre-specified eligibility criteria to answer a specific research question. It uses explicit, systematic methods to minimize bias in the identification, selection, synthesis, and summary of studies. When done well, this provides reliable findings from which conclusions can be drawn and decisions made.

The key characteristics of a systematic review are:
- A clearly stated set of objectives with an explicit, reproducible methodology.
- A systematic search that attempts to identify all studies that would meet the eligibility criteria.
- An assessment of the validity of the findings of the included studies (e.g, assessment of risk of bias and confidence in cumulative estimates).
- Systematic presentation, and synthesis, of the characteristics and findings of the included studies."

Meta-analysis

"Meta-analysis is the use of statistical techniques to combine and summarize the results of multiple studies; they may or may be contained within a systematic review. By combining data from several studies, meta-analyses can provide more precise estimates of the effects of health care than those derived from the individual studies."

Distinction Between Review, an Overview and Meta-analysis by David Sackett

- Review: The general term for all attempts to synthesize the results and conclusions of two or more publications on a given topic.

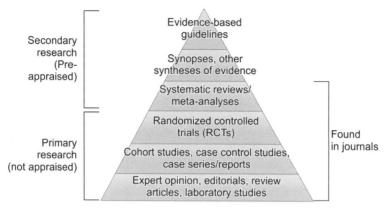

Figure 27.1: Levels of evidence-systematic review.

- Overview: When a review strives to comprehensively identify and track down all the literature on a given topic (also called "systematic literature review").
- Meta-analysis: A specific statistical strategy for assembling the results of several studies into a single estimate.

Figure 27.1 shows the place where the systematic review lies in the hierarchy of level of evidence (Haynes 2006). According to DL Sackett levels of evidence (1996) systematic reviews are considered as level I evidence. [Level I-Systematic reviews, meta-analyses, randomized controlled trials; Level II-Two groups, nonrandomized studies (e.g. cohort, case-control); Level III-One group, nonrandomized (e.g. before and after, pretest and posttest); Level IV-Descriptive studies that include analysis of outcomes (single-subject design, case series); Level V-Case reports and expert opinion that include narrative literature reviews and consensus statements].

STEPS IN A SYSTEMATIC REVIEW (FIG. 27.2)

Developing a systematic review requires a number of discrete steps:

1. Defining an appropriate question

The first step is defining the question for a systematic review. It requires a clear statement of the intervention of interest, relevant patient population and appropriate outcomes. The objectives of the review should be logically derived from the question and be clearly stated. Various methods are used to filter out the words mentioned

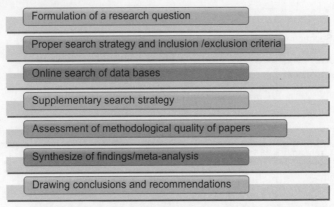

Figure 27.2: Steps in systematic review and meta-analysis.

in the question to trace and extract the relevant information from research articles (E.g. PICO method). The intend in the question should match the words that are being used for the search of research information in the pool of studies to define an appropriate question. For example: The PICO method (CEBM, 2014) can be used to collect evidence from the existing literature by extracting information on the four major components of the systematic review question

2. Searching the literature

The published and unpublished literature should be carefully searched for all reports of appropriate and relevant studies. In systematic reviews of treatment and preventive interventions, randomized comparative trials are generally used as they are considered to be studied with least amount of bias. The search must be as comprehensive as possible to include all the possible searches like electronic, hand, etc., not to miss out any information. Access should include a possible wide number of electronic databases from both English and non-English sources. Proper keyword should be used for search as mentioned in the previous section on designing question (e.g. the keyword 'stroke' used for the search). In an exploratory study analyzing the search strategy for systematic reviews indicate that to guarantee adequate and efficient coverage reviews should search at least Embase, MEDLINE, Web of Science core collection and Google Scholar. Equally appropriate search syntax should be used.

For example: The mainstream health electronic databases which are searched online: Embase, Google Scholar, Web of Science core collection, MEDLINE, Cumulative Index to Nursing and Allied Health Literature (CINAHL), Cochrane Library Database of Systematic Reviews and Physiotherapy Evidence Database (PEDro). However, the search is not limited to these databases alone.

3. Selecting the studies for inclusion in the review

Based on the criterion that has been set to filter out studies like RCTs, prospective studies, population characteristics, etc., the reviewer should describe in the write ups as to how the studies were identified, duplicates were removed, screened for relevance on title, abstract then full text article. In the next step, e.g. in an intervention based review, the type of intervention, population, and outcome are used to create a set of inclusion criteria for studies to be included in the review. The studies identified by the search strategy are then assessed against these criteria to determine if they should be included in the review. To avoid bias, it is important to use a systematic and standardized approach to the appraisal of studies. Ideally, selection of studies should be made by at least two people working independently.

For example: The titles and abstracts of the articles generated by the search strategy were first screened to eliminate irrelevant articles. For the remaining papers, firstly the abstract and finally the full text should be reviewed to determine eligibility.

4. Assessing and reporting the quality of included studies

Assessing the quality of studies form an important part of the systematic review. Once all possible relevant studies have been selected, study quality or validity of the included studies is commented on using the criteria set for quality assessment. A good quality systematic review will comment on all the important study appraisal criteria outlined in the checklist for the studies. Quality assessments are the process of data extraction in systematic reviews and form the basis for data analysis in the next stage of the process. Data extraction forms tailored to various study designs selected for the review should be designed by the reviewer. Extracted data are primarily in numeric values for various criteria in the selected studies like publication in peer reviewed journal, design, randomization, blinding, sample size estimation, etc. Various standardized assessment scales are available for assessing different types of studies. Few types of design studies and the related assessment scales are mentioned within the brackets - For experimental models (CAMARADES), RCTs (STROBE), Diagnostic criteria (STARD), Clinical trials (CONSORT), etc. Readers can refer to Equator network website (www.equator-network.org) to know more about the scales containing checklists for assessing the quality of papers in various types of review.

Example:
In studies involving Physiotherapy interventions, The PEDro scale is a major checklist for assessing the quality of studies. In PEDro rating scale, score of each selected study, which is an indicator of the methodological quality are mentioned as (9-10 = excellent; 6-8 = good; 4-5 = fair; 4 = poor), could be used. The Jadad scale also can be used as an indicator of the methodological quality.

PEDro Rating Criteria:

• Eligibility criteria specified	• Therapist blinding
• Subjects randomly allocated to group	• Assessor blinding
	• Less than 15% drop out rate
• Allocation concealed	• Between group statistical
• Group similar at baseline	comparison reported
• Subject blinding	• Point estimate and variability measure reported

5. Combining the results
Combining and collating the generated data in a systematic review relates to data analysis stage in research. The review should contain information on the steps followed in extracting the data and how the reviewer handled the data. Where appropriate, findings from the individual included studies can then be aggregated to produce a summary estimate or magnitude of effect, odds ratio, P values of the overall effect of the intervention in case of intervention studies. In case of observational studies, a standardized mean difference, weighted mean difference or normalized mean difference. These averages or summary effect forms the basis guidelines on the subject of interest. Sometimes this aggregation is qualitative, but more usually it is a quantitative value from meta-analysis.

Meta-analysis should only be performed when the studies are similar with respect to population, outcome and intervention. A meta-analysis is a two-stage process.

i. The first stage: It is the extraction of data from each individual study and the calculation of a result for each individual study (the "point estimate" or "summary statistic") with an estimate of the chance variation (the "confidence interval").

ii. The second stage: It involves deciding whether it is appropriate to calculate a pooled average result across studies and, if so, calculating and presenting such a result. Part of this process is to give greater weight to the results from studies that give us more information, because these are likely to be closer to the truth we are trying to estimate. In other words a meta-analysis result is to be seen as data from many small set collections of large pool of samples which are otherwise difficult to collect from a single study. Additionally, meta-analysis in a systematic review informs about the heterogeneity or variation as the data is from samples with variations.

The usual way of displaying data from a meta-analysis is by pictorial representation known as a forest plot and a summary measure of effect size with a confidence interval, shown at the bottom of the plot.

6. Placing the findings in context

A systematic review discussion should address the issues such as the quality and heterogeneity, i.e. the variation between studies in the effect of treatment of the included studies, the likely impact of bias and chance, and the applicability of the findings.

KEY CHARACTERISTICS IN DEVELOPMENT OF A SYSTEMATIC REVIEW

In summary, the key characteristics in the development of a systematic review are:

- Clearly stated title and objective for the review.
- Comprehensive strategy to search for studies that address the objectives of the review (relevant studies) that include published and unpublished studies.
- Explicit and justified criteria for the inclusion and exclusion of any study.
- Comprehensive list of all studies identified.

- Comprehensive list of all studies excluded and justification for exclusion.
- Clear presentation of the characteristics of each study included and an analysis of methodological quality.
- Clear analysis of the results of the eligible studies using statistical synthesis of data (meta-analysis) if appropriate and possible.
- Structured report of the review clearly stating the aims, describing the methods and materials and reporting the results.

SYSTEMATIC REVIEW PRESENTATION IN RESEARCH

The subsequent section below detail about the reporting of systematic review findings and major guidelines recommendation (PRISMA) is also mentioned. Reporting of findings of systematic review by an author or authors forms the basis for the synthesis of evidence to be presented to the intended audience. The synthesis must reflect the strength of the findings in relation to the *types of study design (Level)* and the *methodological weaknesses present (biases and study limitations)*. Although there can be study limitations at all levels, please keep in mind that results from a Level I, II, or III study will provide stronger evidence than results from Levels IV or V. To present the results of the synthesis of articles in a systemic review the authors should include the following things in their presentation.

1. Flow diagram
2. Risk of bias table
3. Summary of evidence table
4. Funnel plot
5. Forest plot.

1. Flow diagram

The flow diagram depicts the flow of information through the different phases of a systematic review. It schematically represents out the number of records identified, included and excluded, and the reasons for exclusions. And as much as possible, every step that was followed must be included in the report to eliminate bias and make information as reliable as possible (Fig. 27.3).

2. Risk of bias table

A bias is a systematic error, or deviation from the truth, in results or inferences. Different biases can lead to underestimation or overestimation of the true intervention effect. Differences in risks of

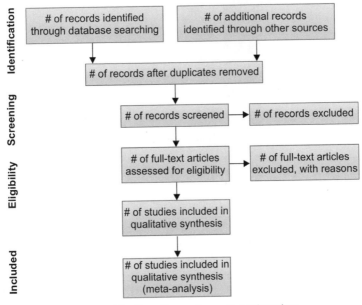

Figure 27.3: Flow diagram in a systematic review.

[From "Preferred Reporting Items for Systematic Reviews and Meta-Analyses: The PRISMA Statement," by D.Moher, A. Liberati, J. Tetzlaff, D. G. Altman; The PRISMA Group, 2009, PLoSMed6(6):e1000097.http://dx.doi.org/10.1371/journal.pmed1000097]

bias can help explain variation in the results of the studies included in a systematic review (i.e. can explain heterogeneity of results). It is important to assess all possible risks of bias in all studies in a review on the domains given in the Table 27.1. [Chapter 8 of the Cochrane Handbook for the most up to date version of the Risk of Bias Tool].

3. Summary of evidence table

Summary of evidence table is the detailed description of individual study characteristics and presenting them in this way would help in understand and relate information in a better way. The inclusion of Summary of findings or Summary of evidence tables in systematic reviews is recommended by publications such as the Cochrane Handbook of Systematic Reviews of Interventions and the Grading of Recommendations Assessment, Development, and Evaluation (GRADE) Working Group guidelines.

Table 27.1: Risk of bias table

Citation	Selection Bias		Performance Bias	Blinding of Outcome Assessment (Detection Bias)		Incomplete Outcome Data (Attrition Bias)		Reporting Bias
	Random Sequence Generation	Allocation Concealment	Blinding of Participants and Personnel	Patient-Reported Outcomes	All-Cause Mortality	Short Term (2–6 wk)	Long Term (>6 wk)	Selective Reporting
Author x (year)	?	–	+	+	–	?	–	?

["Assessing risk of bias in included studies," by J. P. T. Higgins, D. G. Altman, and J. A. C. Sterne, in *Cochrane Handbook for Systematic Reviews of Interventions* (Version 5.1.0), by J. P. T. Higgins and S. Green (Eds.), March 2011.]

Table 27.2: Summary of evidence table

Please mention Table number and [Title of the table] here				
Author/ Year	Level of Evidence/ Study Design/ Participants/ Inclusion Criteria	Intervention and Control Groups	Outcome Measures	Results
Author x (year)	Level of evidence [Level I, II, etc.] Study design [RCT, systematic review, etc.] N = ___ [older adults, youth, children] ___% male, ___% female M age = ____ Manual therapy intervention group n = X Inclusion Criteria [list]	Intervention [summarize] Control [summarize]	[List measures appropriate to answering the focused question]	[List results of the study appropriate to answering the focused question] [Indicate whether the results are statistically significant.]

Note: [Define abbreviations here; e.g., IADLs = independent activities of daily living; RCT = randomized controlled trial].

4. Funnel plot (Fig. 27.4)

Funnel plot is a scatterplot of treatment effect against a measure of study precision or size. It is used primarily as a visual aid for detecting bias or systematic heterogeneity of studies in systematic review and meta-analysis. The standard error of the effect estimate is often chosen as the measure of study size and plotted on the vertical axis with a reversed scale that places the larger, most powerful studies towards the top. The effect estimates from smaller studies should scatter more widely at the bottom, with the spread narrowing among larger studies. In the absence of bias and between study heterogeneity, the scatter will be due to sampling variation alone and the plot will resemble a symmetrical inverted funnel. A triangle centred on a fixed effect summary estimate and extending 1.96 standard errors either side will include about 95% of studies, if no bias is present and the fixed effect assumption (that the true treatment effect is the same in each study) is valid.

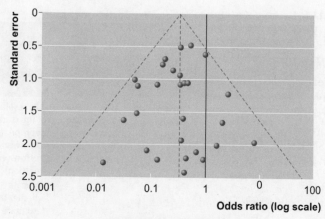

Figure 27.4: Funnel plot.

A symmetric inverted **funnel** shape arises from a 'well-behaved' data set, in which publication bias is unlikely. Possible sources of asymmetry in funnel plots (Egger et al 1997) could be due to:

1. Reporting biases
   a. Publication bias: Delayed publication bias Location biases (e.g. language bias, citation bias, multiple publication bias)
   b. Selective outcome reporting
   c. Selective analysis reporting.
2. Poor methodological quality leading to spuriously inflated effects in smaller studies
   a. Poor methodological design
   b. Inadequate analysis
   c. Fraudulent data and analysis.
3. True heterogeneity
   Size of effect differs according to study size.
4. Artefactual
   In some circumstances, sampling variation can lead to an association between the intervention effect and its standard error.
5. Chance
   Asymmetry may occur by chance, which motivates the use of asymmetry tests.

5. Forest plot

A forest plot (blobbogram) is a graphical display of estimated results from a number of scientific studies addressing the same question, along with the overall results in a systematic review. A sample forest plot depicting the estimate of individual studies and pooled estimate of all the studies developed in the review is mentioned in Figure 27.5.

PRISMA PROTOCOL

Preferred Reporting Items for Systematic Reviews and Meta-Analyses protocols (PRISMA-P) [Moher D, Shamseer L, Clarke M, Ghersi D, Liberati A, Petticrew M, Shekelle P, Stewart LA. Preferred Reporting Items for Systematic Review and Meta-Analysis Protocols (PRISMA-P) 2015 statement. Syst Rev. 2015;4(1):1. doi: 10.1186/2046-4053-4-1]

Protocol
"In the context of systematic reviews and meta-analyses, a protocol is a document that presents an explicit plan."

Preferred Reporting Items for Systematic Reviews and Meta-Analyses (PRISMA) guidelines as a basis for systematic reviews. Please refer to http://www.prismastatement.org/PRISMAStatement/Default.aspx for details on the PRISMA guidelines. The PRISMA checklist is available at http://www.prisma-statement.org/PRISMAStatement/Checklist.aspx. PRISMA guidelines or protocol was developed jointly by Oxford University and Ottawa Hospital Research Institute for transparency in reporting. Ideally, systematic reviews are based on pre-defined

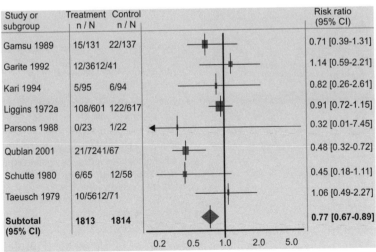

Figure 27.5: Forest plot of a systematic review.

eligibility criteria and conducted according to a pre-defined methodological approach as outlined in an associated protocol.PRISMA-P was
published in 2015 aiming to facilitate the development and reporting
of systematic review protocols. The final PRISMA-P 2015 checklist
contains 17 numbered items (26 including sub-items) Items are
categorized into three main sections: administrative information,
introduction, and methods.

Table 27.3: PRISMA-P 2015 checklist

PRISMA-P (Preferred Reporting Items for Systematic review and Meta-Analysis Protocols) 2015 checklist: recommended items to address in a systematic review protocol* Section and topic	Item No	Checklist item
ADMINISTRATIVE INFORMATION		
Title:		
Identification	1a	Identify the report as a protocol of a systematic review
Update	1b	If the protocol is for an update of a previous systematic review, identify as such
Registration	2	If registered, provide the name of the registry (such as PROSPERO) and registration number
Authors:		
Contact	3a	Provide name, institutional affiliation, e-mail address of all protocol authors; provide physical mailing address of corresponding author
Contributions	3b	Describe contributions of protocol authors and identify the guarantor of the review
Amendments	4	If the protocol represents an amendment of a previously completed or published protocol, identify as such and list changes; otherwise, state plan for documenting important protocol amendments
Support:		

Contd...

Contd...

PRISMA-P (Preferred Reporting Items for Systematic review and Meta-Analysis Protocols) 2015 checklist: recommended items to address in a systematic review protocol* Section and topic	Item No	Checklist item
Sources	5a	Indicate sources of financial or other support for the review
Sponsor	5b	Provide name for the review funder and/or sponsor
Role of sponsor or funder	5c	Describe roles of funder(s), sponsor(s), and/or institution(s), if any, in developing the protocol
INTRODUCTION		
Rationale	6	Describe the rationale for the review in the context of what is already known
Objectives	7	Provide an explicit statement of the question(s) the review will address with reference to participants, interventions, comparators, and outcomes (PICO)
METHODS		
Eligibility criteria	8	Specify the study characteristics (such as PICO, study design, setting, time frame) and report characteristics (such as years considered, language, publication status) to be used as criteria for eligibility for the review
Information sources	9	Describe all intended information sources (such as electronic databases, contact with study authors, trial registers or other gray literature sources) with planned dates of coverage
Search strategy	10	Present draft of search strategy to be used for at least one electronic data base, including planned limits, such that it could be repeated
Study records:		
Data management	11a	Describe the mechanism(s) that will be used to manage records and data throughout the review

Contd...

Contd...

PRISMA-P (Preferred Reporting Items for Systematic review and Meta-Analysis Protocols) 2015 checklist: recommended items to address in a systematic review protocol* Section and topic	Item No	Checklist item
Selection process	11b	State the process that will be used for selecting studies (such as two independent reviewers) through each phase of the review (that is, screening, eligibility and inclusion in meta-analysis)
Data collection process	11c	Describe planned method of extracting data from reports (such as piloting forms, done independently, in duplicate), any processes for obtaining and confirming data from investigators
Data items	12	List and define all variables for which data will be sought (such as PICO items, funding sources), any pre-planned data assumptions and simplifications
Outcomes and prioritization	13	List and define all outcomes for which data will be sought, including prioritization of main and additional outcomes, with rationale
Risk of bias in individual studies	14	Describe anticipated methods for assessing risk of bias of individual studies, including whether this will be done at the outcome or study level, or both; state how this information will be used in data synthesis
Data synthesis	15a	Describe criteria under which study data will be quantitatively synthesised
	15b	If data are appropriate for quantitative synthesis, describe planned summary measures, methods of handling data and methods of combining data from studies, including any planned exploration of consistency (such as I2, Kendall's τ)
	15c	Describe any proposed additional analyses (such as sensitivity or subgroup analyses, meta-regression)

Contd...

Contd...

PRISMA-P (Preferred Reporting Items for Systematic review and Meta-Analysis Protocols) 2015 checklist: recommended items to address in a systematic review protocol* Section and topic	Item No	Checklist item
	15d	If quantitative synthesis is not appropriate, describe the type of summary planned
Meta-bias(es)	16	Specify any planned assessment of meta-bias(es) (such as publication bias across studies, selective reporting within studies)
Confidence in cumulative evidence	17	Describe how the strength of the body of evidence will be assessed (such as GRADE)

DIFFERENCE BETWEEN NARRATIVE REVIEW AND SYSTEMATIC REVIEW

Table 27.4: Difference between narrative review and systematic review

	Classic review or Narrative	Systematic review
Focus of the review	Often addresses a range of issues, bringing these together in an overview. It is the author conclusion from his finding and understanding on the topic of interest	Usually focuses on a single specific question, without trying to provide an overview
Research question	When present, is usually descriptive in nature	Usually explanatory
Search strategy	May be unstated or implicit	Explicit inclusion and exclusion criteria are used
Sources selection	Selective and subject to conscious or unconscious selection bias	Comprehensive, with a deliberate avoidance of selection bias
Types of sources	Mainly published sources, including both theoretical and empirical papers	Published and unpublished ('gray') sources; usually only empirical papers
Quality of sources	Sometimes, and often not according to specified criteria	Always, using specified criteria with focus mainly on methodological issues
Conclusions	Summative conclusions by the author or authors and equally an expert opinion.	Summative or analytical conclusions (meta-analysis)

FURTHER READING

1. "Evidence-Based Medicine: What It Is and What It Isn't," by Sackett DL, Rosenberg WM, Muir Gray JA, Haynes RB, and Richardson WS. British Medical Journal, 1996;312, pp. 71–72.

2. Green BN, Johnson CD, Adams A. Writing narrative literature reviews for peer-reviewed journals: Secrets of the trade. Journal of Chiropratic Medicine, 2006;5, 101-117.

3. Higgins JPT, Green S (Eds). Cochrane Handbook for Systematic Reviews of Interventions Version 5.1.0: updated March 2011. The Cochrane Collaboration; 2011. Available from [www.cochrane-handbook.org]

4. Institute of Medicine. In Finding What Works in Health Care: Standards for Systematic Reviews. Edited by Eden J, Levit L, Berg A, Morton S. Washington, DC: The National Academies Press; 2011.

5. Khan KS, Kunz R, Kleijnen J, Antes G. Systematic Reviews to Support Evidence-Based Medicine. How to Review and Apply findings of Health Care Research. London: RSM Press, 2003.

6. Ma B, Guo J, Qi G, Li H, Peng J, Zhang Y, et al. Epidemiology, quality and reporting characteristics of systematic reviews of traditional Chinese medicine interventions published in Chinese journals. PLoS ONE 2011, 6(5):e20185.

7. Moher D, Shamseer L, Clarke M, Ghersi D, Liberati A, Petticrew M, et al. Preferred Reporting Items for Systematic Review and Meta-Analysis Protocols (PRISMA-P) 2015 statement. Syst Rev. 2015;4(1):1. doi: 10.1186/2046-4053-4-1.

8. Moher D, Tetzlaff J, Tricco AC, Sampson M, Altman DG. Epidemiology and reporting characteristics of systematic reviews. PLoS Med 2007, 4(3):e78.

9. Mulrow CD. Rationale for systematic reviews. In: Chalmers I, Altman DG eds, Systematic Reviews. BMJ Publishing Group, London: 1995;1-8.

10. Shamseer L, Moher D, Clarke M, Ghersi D, Liberati A, Petticrew M, et al. The PRISMA-P Group. Preferred Reporting Items for Systematic Review and Meta-Analysis Protocols (PRISMA-P) 2015: elaboration and explanation. BMJ 2015.349:g7647. doi: 10.1136/bmj.g7647.

11. Sterne Jonathan AC, Sutton Alex J, Ioannidis John PA, Terrin Norma, Jones David R, Lau Joseph, et al. Recommendations for examining and interpreting funnel plot asymmetry in meta-analyses of randomised controlled trials. BMJ 2011;343:d4002.

Journal Club

JOURNAL CLUB

Journal clubs are educational meetings where individuals meet regularly to critically evaluate recent articles in scientific literature. They have often been cited as bridge between research and practice as they encourage application of research in practice. Presenting a scientific paper for a target audience and critically evaluating and justifying whether the ideas and methods used by the author are valid. Journal club presentation is not simply mentioning or reiterating what authors have said. Traditionally journal club aimed to improve critical reading and reviewing the literature in order to improve patient care.

"It is astonishing with how little reading a doctor can practice medicine, but it is not astonishing how badly he may do it."

—Sir William Osler.

Journal clubs have been used as a teaching format in academic medicine for over a hundred years. While their origin is believed by some to have occurred in Europe in the mid 1880s, Sir William Osler is most often recognized as the founder. He began this tradition in North America at McGill University in 1875. Providing its members with up-to-date medical literature was a major focus of journal clubs in the 1960s and 1970s. More recently, in postgraduate medical education, journal clubs have become a forum to teach its members critical appraisal techniques thereby enriching their understanding of the medical literature. They also have emerged as a method to promote the practice of evidence-based medicine.

Moreover journal club can improve the practitioner's educational outcomes and promote lifelong competence in practice-based learning.

Journal club may act as a well-recognized education tool for postgraduate health education programs. It helps them to learn critical analytic skills of available evidences and keep up to date with the development of current medical practices.

Most Journal clubs meet monthly or weekly in places ranged from conference rooms, faculty homes, restaurants, or in the hospital. Most Journal clubs lasted between 1 and 2 hours and reviewed 1-4 articles had 3-4 faculty members present during discussion.

Although the majority of the participants have minimal background training in biostatistics or research the faculty provided formal teaching of critical appraisal skills, clinical epidemiology, and biostatistics in the form of supplemental sessions or hand-outs regarding such methods.

PURPOSE OF JOURNAL CLUB

They are long been recognized as a means of promoting evidence-based medicine and critical appraisal skills. Reading current medical literature (Initiates additional reading). The primary goal of journal club is for keeping up to date with the current literature and the dissemination of information. Journal clubs serves another purpose in the dissemination of information in the practice of evidence-based medicine.

- Critical review of available evidence for its external validity (generalizability).
- Finding the best available evidence for practice application.
- To improve clinical knowledge in a particular area of interest.
- Research projects could be developed from journal club reviews.

STRUCTURE OF RUNNING JOURNAL CLUB

The articles for review are chosen two to three weeks prior to the meeting by a group of expert members of the journal club based on the identification of a clinical problem. Distribution of articles to participants two weeks before meeting is mandatory. The presenting member meet faculty to discuss and critically evaluate the article. Issues of study design and data analysis, as well as the validity and clinical utility of the research findings, are discussed. Selecting articles with opposing hypotheses, results, or conclusions

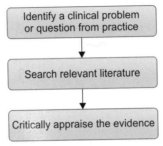

Figure 28.1: Structure of journal club.

or emphasizing different aspects of experimental design (creating a controversy-utilising debate format) on a same subject matter may force participants to show interest as it affects their clinical decisions. Selecting classic articles, analysis of a single article or choosing a problem-based learning method in journal club may improve critical analysis skills of the participants.

CHARACTERISTICS OF SUCCESSFUL JOURNAL CLUBS

- Regular and anticipated meetings to keep the rhythm of the journal club.
- Mandatory attendance, food and emphasize on original research article.
- Clear long- and short-term purpose (explicit written learning objectives).
- Appropriate and convenient meeting timing, and incentives.
- A trained journal club leader to select papers and lead the discussion of the club.
- Circulating papers prior to the meeting.
- A formalized meeting structure and process.
- Using the internet for wider dissemination and data storage.
- Using established critical appraisal processes (structured review checklist).
- Summarizing journal club findings.

HOW TO START (ACCORDING TO RUDOLPH P VALENTINI 1997)

There are no single ideal format for starting a Journal club. However following information from a variety of sources and from our own experiences might help the reader in understanding the formal design of a club.

1. Select a director

The most important step is to select a person who is committed to its organization. A designated leader correlated significantly with effectiveness in one study. This director can be either a faculty member or a chief resident. More importantly, this person must be someone with both a strong interest in resident education and a belief that the journal club plays an important role in it.

2. Define the goals

Preference to teaching of critical appraisal to the participants and keeping them up-to-date with the medical literatures are the main goals of a journal club. The content of the articles selected will be based on these goals. For the programs aiming to keep the participants up to date with the literature, many a times discussing several articles per session or discussing review articles are the common strategies that are followed. The programs interested to teach critical appraisal techniques, are more likely to select fewer articles per session and discuss issues regarding methods and study design.

3. Optimise attendance

Scheduling journal club at a time convenient to the busy schedule of the participants and faculty is often very difficult to achieve but very important.

4. Emphasize the importance of journal club

Selection of relevant articles and interesting topics may encourage audience to participate in the meeting. Moreover the discussion of complex and controversial issues for current practice may attract more numbers.

5. Generate resident interest and enthusiasm in an interactive setting

In general the journal club requires enough audience participation to best educate its participants. It is the constant exchange of ideas and interactions amongst members that help to optimize its teaching potential.

6. Consider creating a curriculum to teach techniques in the critical appraisal of the medical literature

The journal club programs aiming to teach critical appraisal techniques to audience may include some type of formal teaching of these techniques, either as a supplemental lecture series or by devoting some journal club sessions to the analysis of articles illustrating fundamental principles of biostatistics and research methods.

JOURNAL CLUB PRESENTATION

Presentation of the new information is equally important so that the participant gets the right kind of information. The journal club presentation has three parts:
1. Background information and context (author's view)
2. Aims, methods, results, and conclusions (author's view)
3. Presenter's assessment and conclusions (presenter's view).

Presenting Data

The presenter needs to redraw the results to emphasize the major points of the articles, e.g. Redrawn figure, simplified a table or figure, removing the unnecessary data, removing redundant points or using visuals to make the important points. Finally, the applicability of the research findings in the intended situations.

PowerPoint Presentations (Table 28.1)

Presentation should be short and concise covering all the relevant findings in the topic of interest so that a take home message is learnt or given for every member. A sample time management would be, Plan for 30 minutes: roughly 20–25 minutes of talk with slides, and 5+ minutes of questions and discussion
Author's conclusions in 1–3 bullet points
Make figures large enough to read.

Table 28.1: Format for journal article PowerPoint presentation

1. Title slide (1 slide)
  a. Article title
  b. Author
  c. Name of the presenter
2. Introduction (1–2 slides)
  a. Purpose of research
  b. Summary of research
3. Review of Literature (1–2 slides)
  a. List the names of 3–5 articles that were cited by the authors in your journal article
  b. 1–2 sentences describing the importance of each
4. Problem/Hypothesis (1–2 slides)
  a. What problem was the experimenter trying to solve?
  b. What was his or her hypothesis?
	5. Methods (4–6 slides)
	  a. Materials – people used (ages, numbers, characteristics) or other materials
	  b. Experimental and control groups
	  c. Steps used to carry out the experiment
	6. Data (4–6 slides)
	  a. Charts, Graphs, pictures, etc.
	  b. Tables
	7. Discussion (2–4 slides)
	  a. Analysis of the data
	  b. What did the data show
	8. Conclusion (1–2 slides)
	  a. Was the hypothesis correct?
	  b. Is there future research planned?

Timing and Rehearsals

When the presenter is talking, time goes much more slowly for the audience sitting passively in a dimly lit room. So a session goes beyond the allotted time frame the audience begins to get annoyed. Hence the presenter should stick to the allotted time which can be achieved by vigorous rehearsals beforehand.

Question Answer Session

The presenter should be able to answer questions about the research paper, including background, methods, content, conclusions, etc. Answers should be direct, and as short as possible.

Group Presentations

It is essential to practice as a group to ensure that timing and coordination is correct when a journal club presentation done as a group.

JOURNAL CLUB TIPS FOR PRESENTERS (HOW TO GIVE A GOOD JOURNAL CLUB PRESENTATION)

- Identify the problem and place it in scientific context.
- Choose an interesting paper with presentable data, a research paper, not a review.
- Beware of Power Point, Avoid excessive text and avoid reading text to the audience and use a minimum of slides.
- Practice and rehearse the presentation with a timer.
- Don't use a figure unless intended to explain the figure in detail as it takes the audience a long time to assimilate a figure.
- Take Home Message should be achieved for the audience at the end of the meeting.
- Never assume that the audience would have understood the technique as they are thinking and listening, where required, always explain the contents and concepts from basics.
- Make sure visuals are easy to see - enlarge the figures and tables.

There are a few things (Psychological aspects) for the presenter to keep in mind. They are:

- The attending faculty members are not present to judge the presenter, they are there because they find the paper interesting.
- The presenter not expected to be an expert in this area but expected to put in a sincere and determined effort.

- Don't take comments personally. It is not presenter's work, just presenting it.
- An active discussion in the meeting means that the audience is engaged, play the devil's advocate role and defend the authors but no need to oblige the author.

EVALUATION OF THE JOURNAL CLUB

Finally to improve the quality of the Journal club. critical evaluation of the club is essential. To evaluate the outcome of journal club success and performance periodic written surveys should be done:

- To assess the goals and overall satisfaction of participants of the journal club
- To decide whether a change in meeting time and duration of journal club may improve attendance
- To evaluate the knowledge gained by participants.

FURTHER READING

1. Cave MT, Clandinin DJ. Revisiting the journal club. Medical Teacher 2007;29(4):365-70.
2. Deenadayalan, Y, Grimmer-Somers K, Prior M, Kumar S. How to run an effective journal club: a systematic review. Journal of Evaluation in Clinical Practice, 2008;14: 898–911. doi:10.1111/j.1365-2753.2008.01050.
3. Jeanne St Pierre. Changing Nursing Practice Through a Nursing Journal Club. Medsurg Nursing; Pitman Vol. 14, Iss. 6, 2005;390-2.
4. Lee AG, et al. Using the Journal Club to Teach and Assess Competence in Practice-based Learning and Improvement: A Literature Review and Recommendation for Implementation. Survey of Ophthalmology 2005;50(6):542-48.
5. Mark D. Schwartz, Deborah Dowell, Jaclyn Aperi, Adina Kalet. Improving journal club presentations, or, I can present that paper in under 10 minutes. ACP J Club. 2007;147:A8. doi: 10.7326/ACPJC-2007-147-1-A08.
6. R. Brian Haynes. The origins and aspirations of ACP Journal Club. ACP J Club. 1991;114:A18. doi: 10.7326/ACPJC-1991-114-1-A18.
7. Sidorov J. How are internal medicine residency journal clubs organized, and what makes them successful? Arch Intern Med 1995;155(11):1193-97.
8. Spillane AJ, Crowe PJ. The role of the journal club in surgical training. Australian and New Zealand Journal of Surgery, 1998;68:288–291. doi:10.1111/j.1445-2197.1998.tb02085.

Glossary

Abstract
A brief summary of the research report from researcher.

Allocation Concealment
In a randomized clinical trial, the inability of the individual making the assignment to predict the group to which the next individual will be assigned.

Allocation Ratio
In a randomized clinical trial the proportion of participants intended for each study and control group.

Alpha Level
A specific probability level depicted as 'α', set in advance in research to indicate what the researcher considers significant; typically set at .05.

Alternative Hypothesis
In statistical significance testing, the actual choices are between the null hypothesis and an alternative hypothesis. The alternative hypothesis states that a difference or association exists.

Analysis of Covariance (ANCOVA)
It is a statistical procedure for analysis of data that contains a continuous dependent variable and a mixture of nominal and continuous independent variables.

Analysis of Variance (ANOVA)
Anova is a statistical test to identify whether there are any significant differences between three or more simple means. It is a statistical procedure for analysis of data that contains a continuous dependent variable and more than one nominal independent variable. ANOVA procedures include one-way and factorial ANOVA.

Applied Research

Research conducted to address a practical problem to suggest solutions.

Bar Graph (Histogram)

It is a graphic display of the scores in a frequency distribution (vertical or horizontal bars).

Bivariable Analysis

Statistical analysis in which there is one dependent variable and one independent variable.

Bonferroni Test

A post hoc test that adjusts for experiment wise error by dividing the alpha value by the total number of tests performed.

Ceiling Effect

Failure of a dependent measure to detect a difference because it was too easy.

Central Tendency

A single number or value that describes the typical or central score among a set of scores.

Chi-square Test

A non-parametric test that compares between two or more samples on the observed frequency of values with the expected frequency of values.

Closed-ended Question

In questionnaires and interviews, a question that presents the respondent with a limited number of alternatives to select.

Cluster Sampling

A method of sampling in which clusters of individuals are identified, sampled, and then all individuals in each cluster are included in the sample.

Cohort

A group of people born at about the same time and exposed to the same societal events; cohort effects are confounded with age in a cross-sectional study.

Concurrent Validity

This describes the extent to which a test distinguishes between the different samples it should be expected to distinguish between. This is usually determined by comparing the test with an external gold standard.

Confidence Interval/Interval Estimate (95%)

In statistical terms, the interval of numerical values within which one can be 95% confident that the value being estimated lies.

Confidence Limits

These are the upper and lower extremes of the confidence interval.

Confounding

Failure to control for the effects of a third variable in an experimental design.

Content Validity

This describes the extent to which the variables or items (e.g. temperature) being measured by a test (e.g. thermometer) are related to that which should be measured by such a test.

Continuous Data

A type of data with an unlimited number of equally spaced potential values (e.g. diastolic blood pressure, cholesterol).

Convergent Validity

Convergent validity describes the extent of correlation between results from a test with results obtained from other similar tests, that is, when applied simultaneously, similar tests measuring the same variables ought to show a correlation in their respective results.

Correlation Analysis

It is a statistical procedure that is used to estimate the strength of the relationship between a continuous dependent variable and a continuous independent variable when both the dependent variable and the independent variable are selected by naturalistic sampling.

Correlation Coefficient

It is an estimate of the strength of the association between a dependent variable and an independent variable when both are obtained using naturalistic sampling (e.g. Pearson's and Spearman's correlation coefficients).

Criterion Validity

An umbrella term used in epidemiology encompassing predictive, concurrent, convergent and discriminant validity.

Cross-Over Study

A type of paired design in which the same individual receives a study and a control therapy, and an outcome is assessed for each therapy.

Cross-Sectional Study

It is a study that identifies individuals with and without the condition or disease under study and the characteristic or exposure of interest at the same point in time. A cross-sectional study may be regarded as a special type of case-control study.

Cross-Validity

Describes the stability of a test's validity when applied to different subgroups of a target population.

Degrees of Freedom

The number of values in a study that have the freedom to vary, given a mathematical restriction that needs to be put in place when estimating one statistic from an estimate of another.

Discrete Data

A kind of data with a limited number of categories or potential values. It may be further classified as either nominal or ordinal data.

Discriminant Validity

Discriminant validity describes the extent to which the results of a test are dissimilar from the results of another unrelated test, that is, when applied simultaneously, dissimilar tests that do not measure similar properties should not show a correlation in their respective results.

Dispersion

Spread of data around a measure of central tendency, such as a mean.

Distribution

It is the frequencies or relative frequencies of all possible values of a characteristic.

Effect Size

It is a measure of the magnitude of the difference or association found in the sample.

Effectiveness

Effectiveness is the extent to which a treatment produces a beneficial effect when implemented under the usual conditions of clinical care for a particular group of patients. In the context of cost-effectiveness, effectiveness incorporates desirable outcomes and undesirable outcomes, and may be referred to as net effectiveness.

Efficacy

Efficacy is the extent to which a treatment produces a beneficial effect when assessed under the ideal conditions of an investigation or a study.

Ethnography

Field observation in which the researcher spends an extended period of time in the natural setting of a social group to document their customs, habits, and actions.

Experimental Method

A method of determining whether variables are related in which the researcher manipulates the independent variable and controls all other variables either by randomization or by direct experimental control.

Experimenter Bias

Any intentional or unintentional influence that the experimenter exerts on subjects to confirm the hypothesis under investigation.

External Validity (Generalizability)

This describes the extent to which results from a study can be generalized to a wider population.

Face Validity

This describes the extent to which a test appears to be measuring what it purports to measure, on inspection. Face validity is a weak type of validity because it is based on subjective judgments.

Factor Analysis

It is a method for modeling observed variables, and their covariance structure, in terms of a smaller number of underlying unobservable latent factors. It is used to reduce a large number of variables into fewer numbers of factors. This technique extracts maximum common variance from all variables and puts them into a common score.

Fisher's Exact Procedure

A method for calculating P values for data with one nominal dependent variable and one nominal independent variable when any of the frequencies predicted by the null hypothesis are less than 5.

Frequency Polygon

A graphic display of a frequency distribution in which the frequency of each score is plotted on the vertical axis, with the plotted points connected by straight lines.

Gaussian Distribution

A distribution of data assumed in many statistical procedures. The Gaussian distribution is a symmetrical, continuous, bell-shaped curve with its mean value corresponding to the highest point on the curve. (Synonym: normal distribution).

Homogeneous

When used in the context of a meta-analysis, homogeneous refers to investigations which can be combined into a single meta-analysis because the study characteristics being examined do not substantially affect the outcome.

Incremental Validity

Incremental validity compares a test with other related tests regarding the best reflection of a measured property.

Independent Variable

The variable that is manipulated to observe its effect on the dependent variable.

Inferential Statistics

Statistics designed to determine whether results based on sample data are generalizable to a population.

Informed Consent

In research ethics, the principle that participants in a study be informed in advance of all aspects of the research that may influence their decision to participate.

Institutional Review Board (IRB)

An ethics review committee established to review research proposals. The IRB is composed of scientists, non-scientists, and legal experts.

Intention to Treat

A method for data analysis in a randomized clinical trial in which individual outcomes are analyzed according to the group to which they have been randomized even if they never received the treatment to which they were assigned.

Interaction Effect

The differing effect of one independent variable on the dependent variable, depending on the level of another independent variable.

Internal Validity

This describes the extent to which results from a study can be said to reflect the 'true' results when study design and methodology are taken into consideration. In other words, the extent to which test methodology permits reflection of the 'true picture'.

Inter-rater Reliability

It describes the extent of agreement of test results when two or more assessors make simultaneous measurements, for example agreement between judges in gymnastic sporting events.

Interval Scale

A scale of measurement in which the intervals between numbers on the scale are all equal in size.

Main Effect

A term used in factorial ANOVA to indicate statistical tests used to examine each factor separately. May also refer to the relationship between the independent variable and the dependent variable that reflect the relationship stated in the study hypothesis.

McNemar's Test

A statistical significance test for paired data when there is one nominal dependent variable and one nominal independent variable.

Mean

It is the sum of the measurements divided by the number of measurements being added together (The center of gravity of a distribution of observations).

Median

It is the mid-point of a distribution. The median is chosen so that half the data values occur above and half occur below the median.

Meta-analysis

A set of statistical procedures for combining the results of a number of studies to provide a general assessment of the relationship between variables.

Mode

A measure of central tendency; the most frequent score in a distribution of scores.

Nominal Data

A type of data with named categories. Nominal data may have more than two categories that cannot be ordered (e.g. race, eye color). Nominal data may have only two categories, i.e. dichotomous data, that can be ordered one above another (e.g. dead/alive).

Nonparametric Statistics

It is the type of statistical procedures that do not make assumptions about the distribution of parameters in the population being sampled. Nonparametric statistical methods are not free of assumptions such as the assumption of random sampling. They are most often used for ordinal data but may be used for continuous data converted to an ordinal scale.

Nonprobability Sampling

A type of sampling procedure in which one cannot specify the probability that any member of the population will be included in the sample.

Null Hypothesis

It is the assertion that no association or difference between the independent variable of interest and the dependent variables exists in the larger population from which the study samples are obtained.

Number Needed to Treat

The number of patients, similar to the study patients, who need to be treated to obtain one fewer bad outcome or one more good outcome compared to the control group treatment.

Observational Study

An investigation in which the assignment is conducted by observing the subjects who meet the inclusion and exclusion criteria. Case-control and cohort studies are observational studies.

Odds

A ratio in which the numerator contains the number of times an event occurs and the denominator contains the number of times the event does not occur.

Odds Ratio

A ratio measuring the strength of an association applicable to all types of studies employing nominal data but is required for case-control and cross-sectional studies. The odds ratio for case-control and cross-sectional studies is measured as the odds of having the risk factor if the condition is present divided by the odds of having the risk factor if the condition is not present.

One-Tailed Test

A statistical significance test in which deviations from the null hypothesis in only one direction are considered. Use of a one-tailed test implies that the investigator does not consider a true deviation in the opposite direction to be possible.

Ordinal Data

A type of data with a limited number of categories and with an inherent ordering of the categories from lowest to highest. Ordinal data, however, say nothing about the spacing between categories (e.g. Spasticity grade 1, 2, 3, and 4).

P Value

The probability of obtaining data at least as extreme as the data obtained in the investigation's sample if the null hypothesis is true. The P value is considered the bottom line in statistical significance testing.

Parameter

It is a value that summarizes the distribution of a large population. One purpose of statistical analysis is to estimate a population's parameter from the sample's observations.

Pilot Study

A small-scale study conducted prior to conducting an actual experiment; designed to test and refine procedures.

Power

It is the ability of an investigation to demonstrate statistical significance when a true association or difference of a specified strength exists in the population being sampled. (Power = 1 - Type II error).

Predictive Validity

This describes the extent to which a test result predicts what it should be logically expected to predict.

Probability

A proportion in which the numerator contains the number of times an event occurs and the denominator includes the number of times an event occurs plus the number of times it does not occur.

Probability Sampling

Type of sampling procedure in which one is able to specify the probability that any member of the population will be included in the sample.

Qualitative Data

Verbal, descriptive data that is typically presented in everyday language without numbers or statistics.

Quantitative Data

Numerical data that is typically reported in tables, figures, and statistics.

Quasi-experimental Design

A type of design that approximates the control features of true experiments to infer that a given treatment had its intended effect.

Quota Sampling

It is a sampling procedure in which the sample is chosen to reflect the numerical composition of various subgroups (e.g. male/female) in the population. A haphazard sampling technique is used to obtain the sample.

Randomization

A method of assignment in which individuals have a known, but not necessarily equal, probability of being assigned to a particular study group or control group.

Range

The difference between the highest and lowest data values in a population or sample.

Ratio Scale

A scale of measurement in which there is an absolute zero point, indicating an absence of the variable being measured.

Regression Equation

A mathematical equation that allows prediction of one behavior when the score on another variable is known.

Relative Risk

It is a ratio of the probability of developing the outcome in a specified period of time if the risk factor is present divided by the probability of developing the outcome in that same period of time if the risk factor is not present. The relative risk is a measure of the strength of association applicable to cohort and randomized clinical trials. In case-control studies, the odds ratio often can be used to approximate the relative risk.

Response Rate

In survey research, the percentage of people who complete the survey.

Robust

A statistical procedure is robust if its assumptions can be violated without substantial effects on its conclusions.

Sampling

The process of choosing members of a population to be included in a sample.

Sampling Bias

A problem when sampling procedures overlook certain categories of people in the population, creating a non-representative sample.

Sampling Distribution

A probability distribution for the values of an inferential statistic, given the assumption that the null hypothesis is true.

Sampling Error

An error introduced by chance differences between the estimate obtained in a sample and the true value in the larger population from which the sample was drawn. Sampling error is inherent in the use of sampling methods and its magnitude is measured by the standard error.

Scientific Method

An approach to gathering knowledge that relies on an objective set of rules for gathering, evaluating, and reporting information.

Self-report Measure

A dependent measure in which participants provide information about themselves, e.g. by filling out a questionnaire or responding to interview questions.

Simple Random Sampling

A sampling procedure in which each member of the population has an equal probability of being included in the sample.

Split-Half Reliability

Describes the extent of agreement of the results from two stable halves of a split test.

Standard Deviation

It is a commonly used measure of the spread or dispersion of data. The standard deviation squared is known as the variance.

Standard Distribution

It is the distributions for which statistical value tables have been developed. Use of standard distributions, when chosen appropriately, simplify the calculation of P values and confidence intervals.

Standard Error

The spread or dispersion of point estimates, such as the mean obtained from all possible samples of a specified size. The standard error is equal to the standard deviation divided by the square root of the sample size (See: sampling error).

Stratified Random Sampling

A sampling procedure in which the population is divided into strata followed by random sampling from each stratum.

Surrogate Endpoint

The use of measurements such as test results instead of clinically important outcome measures to assess the outcomes of an investigation. In order to be an appropriate measure of outcome, surrogate endpoints require a strong association between the surrogate endpoint and a relevant clinical outcome.

Test–Retest Reliability

Describes the extent of agreement of initial test results with results of repeat measurement made later on.

Two-Tailed Test

It is a statistical significance test in which deviations from the null hypothesis in either direction are considered. The use of a two-tailed test implies that the investigator was willing to consider deviations in either direction before data were collected.

Type I Error

An error that occurs when data demonstrate a statistically significant result when no true association or difference exists in the population. The alpha level is the size of the Type I error which will be tolerated (usually 5%).

Type II Error

An error that occurs when the sample's observations fail to demonstrate statistical significance when a true association or difference actually exists in the population. The beta level is the size of the Type II error that will be tolerated.

Validity

The validity of a test describes the extent to which a test actually measures what it purports to measure.

Variable

Generally refers to a characteristic for which measurements are made in a study. A variable is the representation of those measurements in an analysis. Continuous or ordinal scale data are expressed using one variable, as are nominal data with only two categories.

Variance

Variance is the mean square deviation of data from the mean.

Question Bank

QUESTION BANK

1. Define research. Why research is required in Physiotherapy? Explain the difficulties encountered in Physical Therapy Research.
2. What is Research Proposal? Why it is required? Describe a suitable format for Research Proposal.
3. Why a research work should be published? Describe a suitable format to publish a research report in a journal.
4. Define reliability and validity. Explain the methods to assess the reliability and validity of instruments used in experimental research.
5. Define research problem. Describe factors considered in selection of a Research Problem.
6. Describe correlation and regression analysis.
7. Define a questionnaire as research tool. Describe the uses and limitations of questionnaire.
8. Explain the Guidelines for writing research report.
9. Describe various research designs in detail.
10. Describe in detail about different types of sampling methods.
11. Describe the steps in writing a Research Proposal.
12. Define Reliability. Describe the testing Methods to determine the reliability of instruments used in Research Process.
13. Why Publication is required in Research? Write the Components of Journal Research Report?
14. What are the types of error that occur in research? Explain each type with example.
15. Define Research problem and enumerate the factors contribute its selection and techniques.
16. Why the literature review is necessary? What is Primary and Secondary Literature? Explain reviewing process.
17. Describe in detail, the levels of measurement that might be involved in research with appropriate examples.
18. Explain the basic principles of questionnaire design adding a note on its advantages and disadvantages.
19. Methods of presentation of data.

SHORT QUESTIONS

1. A note on type I and type II errors.
2. Advantages and disadvantages of questionnaire method.
3. Attitude scales.
4. Barriers to Research in Physiotherapy.
5. Blinding in research.
6. Case report/study.
7. Clinical and statistical significance.
8. Coefficient of correlation.
9. Components of research problem.
10. Components of research process.
11. Confidence interval.
12. Consent form.
13. Define dependent variable and Independent variable with examples.
14. Define experimental and non- experimental research and its purpose.
15. Define research.
16. Describe in detail the experimental design of research study.
17. Difference between parametric and non-parametric statistics.
18. Discuss the limitation in experimental research.
19. Discuss the process of experimental research.
20. Ethics in research.
21. Experimental and null hypothesis.
22. Experimental validity.
23. Experimental Vs. Non-experimental design.
24. Explain experimental design.
25. Group comparison experimental Research and its limitation.
26. How to formulate a research problem?
27. Hypothesis.
28. Importance of post hoc tests.
29. Importance of research in physical therapy.
30. Internet sites for physiotherapy evidence search.
31. Interpretation of statistical results.
32. Level of measurements.
33. Level of significance.
34. Levels of evidence.
35. Measurement tools.
36. Measures of central tendency.
37. Measures of dispersion.

38. Methods of presentation of the data.
39. Necessity of review of literature.
40. Normal distribution.
41. Parametric versus Non-parametric tests.
42. Pilot study.
43. Population and sample.
44. Presentation of data.
45. Primary and secondary literature.
46. Principle ethics of human research.
47. Principles for human research.
48. Process of experimental research.
49. Quantitative research design.
50. Quasi experimental study.
51. Questionnaire method.
52. Randomization.
53. Rating scales in measurement.
54. RCT research designs.
55. Reliability and validity of data collection tools.
56. Research paradigms.
57. Review of literature.
58. Risk ratio and odds ratio.
59. Sample size determination.
60. Sampling methods in research.
61. Scales of measurements.
62. Sensitivity and specificity.
63. Significance of research proposal.
64. Standard deviation.
65. Testing of hypothesis.
66. Type of errors in a study.
67. Types of correlation.
68. Types of qualitative research.
69. Types of research.
70. What is random sample?
71. Why literature review is required?
72. Purpose of journal club.
73. Structure of journal club.
74. Systematic review.
75. Principles of journal club.
76. Psychometric properties of a tool.

Appendix

Statistical Tests

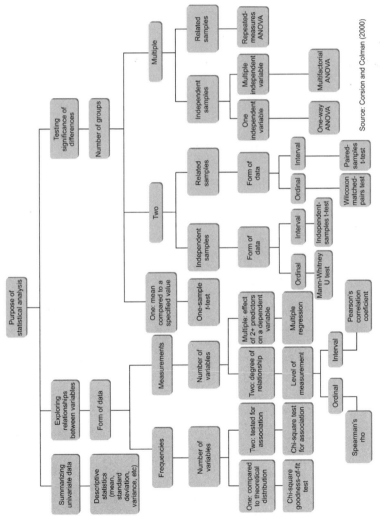

Source: Corsion and Colman (2000)

Statistical Tests in Psychometric Testing

Properties	Statistics	Sample size	Tools	Level of measurements
Test retest reliability	ICC Kappa statistic	30	Primary outcome measure	Repeated measurement
Level of agreement	Bland Altman graph, Standard Error of Measurement, Minimum Detectable change	30	Primary outcome measure	Repeated measurement
Internal consistency	Croanbach's alpha	150+	Primary outcome measure	Once
Scale structure/ Factorial validity	Factor analysis PCA/CFA Structural equation modelling (SEM)	150 + (1 : 10 cases) (150 + 150 for CFA)	Primary outcome measure	Once
Scale construct validity	Multiple regression analysis	150+	Primary outcome measure	Once
Discrimination of items/item total correlation validity	Item analysis (item total correlation validity index >0.2)	150+	Primary outcome measure	Once
Ceiling and floor effect	Skewness index between -1 to $+1$ Or Highest and lowest possible scores not more than 15%	150+	Primary outcome measure	Once
Divergent validity	Pearson/ spearman correlation coefficient	150+ (less sample size also can be considered)	Primary outcome measure + Pain, disability and Qol tools	Once

Properties	Statistics	Sample size	Tools	Level of measurements
Content validity*	Mean or median	30	Rating or likerts scale used*	Once
Criterion validity	Pearson/ Spearman correlation coefficient	Minimum 30 (100+/more preferable)	Any other measure of same kind	Once
Concurrent validity (Criterion is in the present)	Pearson/ Spearman correlation coefficient	Minimum 30 (100+/more preferable)	Gold standard measure	Once
Discriminant validity	Pearson/ Spearman correlation coefficient	Minimum 30 (100+/more preferable)	Other construct scale, e.g. depression	Once
Convergent validity	Pearson/ spearman correlation coefficient	Minimum 30 (100+/more preferable)	Same construct scale	Once
Known group validity	T test/Z test	150+	Primary outcome measure (acute vs chronic)	Once
Responsiveness (sensitivity to change) Internal	T test/Z test Effect size Standard responses mean (SRM)	150+	Primary outcome measure	Repeated measurement (first and 14th day)
Responsiveness External	Receiver operating characteristics/ Area under curve ROC/AUC (Improved vs not improved)	150+	Primary outcome measure + Global perceived effect scale (GPE) or GROC	Once
Prediction power	Cross-sectional and longitudinal multivariate hierarchical regression analysis	150+	Primary outcome measure + Pain, disability and Qol tools	Repeated measurement (first and 14th day)

*1. Content equivalence is assessed under two headings:

   i. Are the words in the translated Tamil version presented fluently and correctly as in the original version? For this answers from 30 expert panel members fall between 'mostly agree' to 'strongly agree' on a 5 or 7-point Likert scale.

   ii. Do the words and phrase in the translated Tamil version have the same semantic meaning compared with the original version? For this answers from 30 expert panel members fall between 'mostly agree' to 'strongly agree' on a 5 or 7-point Likert scale.

2. Content relevance is assessed by asking: How the tamil statement is relevant to assessing disability in patients? For this answers from 30 expert panel members fall between 'mostly agree' to 'strongly agree' on a 5 or 7-point Likert scale.

3. Content representativeness was assessed by asking "How well is the content of the scale is representing the entire domain of assessing the disability of patients?" For this answers from 30 expert panel members falls between 'mostly agree' to 'strongly agree' on a 5 or 7-point Likert scale.

Pie Diagram

Graphical representation of data in a research.

Gender Distribution

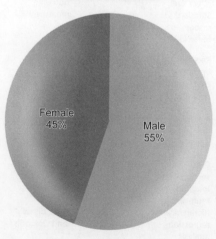

Scatter Diagram

This is a diagrammatic representation of the data of two variables as to how the participated samples are scattered within the values mentioned for the two variables.

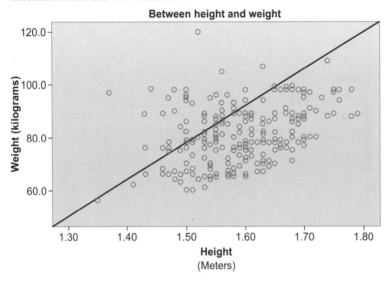

Bar Graph

Diagrammatic representation two variables (Pain and Pain severity) in Bar graph.

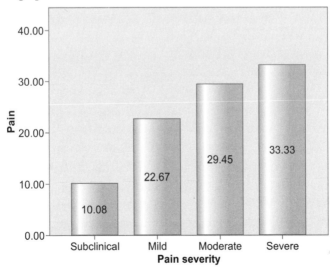

Line Diagram

Diagrammatic representation of two variables in line diagram.

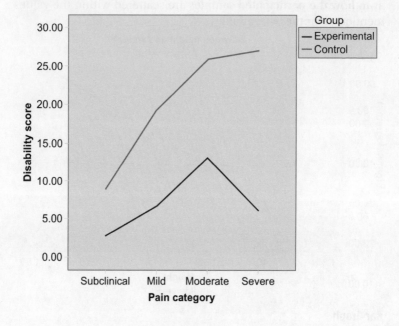

Box Plot

A box plot represents the spread of a variable for each group. The line running in the middle represents the midpoint of all the values.

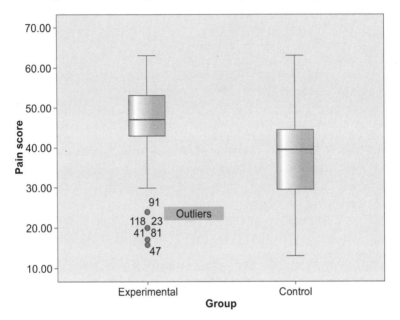

Further Reading

1. Agency for Healthcare Research and Quality (http://www.ahrq. gov/clinic/epcix.htm)
2. Altman DG. Practical Statistics for Medical Research. London: Chapman and Hall, 1991.
3. Andresen EM. "Criteria for assessing the tools of disability outcomes research." Arch Phys Med Rehabil, 2000;81(12 Suppl 2): S15-20.
4. Bangert-Drowns RL. 'The effects of school-based substance abuse education: a meta-analysis'. Journal of Drug Education, 1988;18, 3, 243-65.
5. Bangert RL, Kulik JA, Kulik CC. 'Individualised systems of instruction in secondary schools.' Review of Educational Research, 1983;53, 143-158.
6. Baugh F. 'Correcting effect sizes for score reliability: A reminder that measurement and substantive issues are linked inextricably'. Educational and Psychological Measurement, 2002;62, 2, 254-263.
7. Beaton D, Bombardier C, Guillemin F, Ferraz MB. Recommendations for the cross-cultural adaptation of health status measures. New York: American Academy of Orthopaedic Surgeons. 2002:1-9.
8. Beaton DE, Bombardier C, Guillemin F, Ferraz MB. Guidelines for the process of cross-cultural adaptation of self-report measures. Spine. 2000;25(24):3186-91.
9. Centre for Evidence-Based Medicine (http://www.cebm.net/)
10. Cliff N. 'Dominance Statistics - ordinal analyses to answer ordinal questions' Psychological Bulletin, 1993;114, 3. 494-509.
11. Clinical Evidence (www.clinicalevidence.com)
12. Cochrane Library (www.cochrane.org/)
13. Cohen J. Statistical Power Analysis for the Behavioral Sciences. NY: Academic Press, 1969.
14. Cohen J. 'The Earth is Round (p<.05)'. American Psychologist, 1994;49, 997-1003.
15. Cohen PA, Kulik JA, Kulik CC. 'Educational outcomes of tutoring: a meta-analysis of findings.' American Educational Research Journal, 1982;19, 237-248.

16. Creswell John W. Research Design: Qualitative, Quantitative and Mixed Methods Approaches (2nd edn), Thousand Oaks, CA, Sage, 2003.
17. Currier DP. Elements of Research in Physical Therapy: Williams and Wilkins; 1990.
18. Dillman DA.Mail and internet surveys - the tailored design method, 2nd ed. New York. Wiley, 2007.
19. Domholdt E. Physical Therapy Research: Principles and Applications: Saunders; 1993.
20 Domholdt E. Rehabilitation Research: Principles and Applications: Elsevier Saunders; 2005.
21. Dowson V. "Time of day effects in school-children's immediate and delayed recall of meaningful material". 2000. Report http://www.cem.dur.ac.uk/ebeuk/research/terse/library.htm
22. Earl-Slater Alan. The Handbook of Clinical Trials and Other Research. Radcliffe Publishing Ltd. 2002. ISBN 1-85775-485-9.
23. Effective Medical Writing. Peh WCG and NG K H Singapore Medical Journal 2008;49(7) 522 smj.sma.org.sg/4907/4907emw1.pdf
24. Epstein J, et al. "A review of guidelines for cross-cultural adaptation of questionnaires could not bring out a consensus." Journal of Clinical Epidemiology, 2015;68(4): 435-441.
25. Finn JD, Achilles CM. 'Answers and questions about class size: A statewide experiment.' American Educational Research Journal, 1990;27, 557-577.
26. Fitz-Gibbon CT. 'A Typology of Indicators for an Evaluation-Feedback Approach' in Visscher AJ, Coe R, (Eds.) School Improvement Through Performance Feedback. Lisse: Swets and Zeitlinger, 2002.
27. Fitz-Gibbon CT. 'Meta-analysis: an explication.' British Educational Research Journal, 1984;10, 2, 135-144.
28. Fitzpatrick R, Davey C, et al. "Evaluating patient-based outcome measures for use in clinical trials." Health Technol Assess, 1998; 2(14): i-iv, 1-74.
29. Fleiss JL. 'Measures of Effect Size for Categorical Data' in Cooper H, Hedges LV, (Eds.). The Handbook of Research Synthesis. New York: Russell Sage Foundation, 1994.
30. Fletcher-Flinn CM, Gravatt B. 'The efficacy of Computer Assisted Instruction (CAI): a meta-analysis.' Journal of Educational Computing Research, 1995;12(3), 219-242.

31. Fowler Floyd J. Survey research methods (4th edition). Thousand Oaks, CA: Sage, 2008.
32. Fuchs LS, Fuchs D. 'Effects of systematic formative evaluation: a meta-analysis.' Exceptional Children, 1986;53, 199-208.
33. Giaconia RM, Hedges LV. 'Identifying features of effective open education.' Review of Educational Research, 1982;52, 579-602.
34. Glass GV, McGaw B, Smith ML. Meta-Analysis in Social Research. London: Sage, 1981.
35. Guillemin F, Bombardier C, Beaton D. Cross-cultural adaptation of health-related quality of life measures: literature review and proposed guidelines. Journal of clinical epidemiology. 1993;46(12):1417-32.
36. Guyatt G, Rennie D, Meade MO, Cook DJ. Users' Guides to the Medical Literature: Essentials of Evidence-Based Clinical Practice 3e: McGraw-Hill Education; 2014.
37. Guyatt GH, Sackett DL, Cook DJ. Users' guides to the medical literature. II.How to use an article about therapy or prevention. A. Are the results of thestudy valid? JAMA 1993;270:2598-2601.
38. Guyatt GH, Sackett DL, Cook DJ. Users' guides to the medical literature. II.How to use an article about therapy or prevention. B. What were the results and will they help me in caring for my patients? JAMA 1993;271:59-63.
39. Hagen and Thorndike, Robert. L. eds. *Measurement And Evaluation In Psychology And Education.* New York: John Wiley & Sons, 1977.
40. Harlow LL, Mulaik SS, Steiger JH (Eds).What if there were no significance tests? Mahwah NJ: Erlbaum, 1997.
41. Hedges L, Olkin I. Statistical Methods for Meta-Analysis. New York: Academic Press, 1985.
42. Hembree R. 'Correlates, causes effects and treatment of test anxiety.' Review of Educational Research, 1988;58(1),47-77.
43. Hicks C. Research Methods for Clinical Therapists: Applied Project Design and Analysis: Churchill Livingstone; 1999.
44. How to read and review a scientific journal article. Duke University Writing Studio twp.duke.edu/uploads/media_items/scientificarticlereview.original.pdf
45. How to Read a Paper: The Basics of Evidence-Based Medicine by Trisha Greenhalgh, 2010.
46. How to read a scientific article. Mary Purugganan & Jan Hewitt, Rice University www.owlnet.rice.edu/~cainproj/courses/HowToReadSciArticle.pdf

47. How to read a scientific paper. John W. Little & Roy Parker-University of Arizona www.biochem.arizona.edu/classes/bioc568/papers.htm

48. How to Write a Paper: George M. Hall (2008).

49. http://www.cebm.net/critical-appraisal/

50. https://www.essentialevidenceplus.com/

51. https://www.essentialevidenceplus.com/index.cfm.

52. Huberty CJ. 'A history of effect size indices'. Educational and Psychological Measurement, 2002;62, 2, 227-240.

53. Hyman RB, Feldman HR, Harris RB, Levin RF, Malloy GB. 'The effects of relaxation training on medical symptoms: a meat-analysis.' Nursing Research, 1989;38, 216-220.

54. Jaeschke R, Singer J, Guyatt GH. "Measurement of health status. Ascertaining the minimal clinically important difference". Control Clin Trials. 1989;10 (4): 407–15. PMID 2691207. doi:10.1016/0197-2456(89)90005-6.

55. Jump up Revicki, Dennis. "Recommended methods for determining responsiveness and minimally important difference for patient reported outcomes". Journal of Clinical Epidemiology. 2008;61 (2): 102–109. PMID 18177782. doi:10.1016/j.jclinepi.2007.03.012

56. Kaplan, David (eds). The Sage Handbook of Quantitative Methodology for the Social Sciences,Thousand Oaks, CA, Sage, 2004.

57. Kathleen W. Brown, Paul C. Cozby Daniel W. Kee Research Methods in Human Development; Mayfield Publishing Company; Mountain View, California London. Toronto, 1999.

58. Kavale KA, Forness SR. 'Hyperactivity and diet treatment: a meat-analysis of the Feingold hypothesis.' Journal of Learning Disabilities, 1983;16, 324-330.

59. Keselman HJ, Huberty CJ, Lix LM, Olejnik S, Cribbie RA, Donahue B, Kowalchuk RK, Lowman LL, Petoskey MD, Keselman JC, Levin JR. 'Statistical practices of educational researchers: An analysis of their ANOVA, MANOVA, and ANCOVA analyses'. Review of Educational Research, 1998;68, 3, 350-386.

60. Kirk RE. 'Practical Significance: A concept whose time has come'. Educational and Psychological Measurement, 1996;56, 5, 746-759.

61. Kothari CR. Research Methodology: Methods and Techniques: New Age International (P) Limited; 2004.

62. Kulik JA, Kulik CC, Bangert RL. 'Effects of practice on aptitude and achievement test scores.' American Education Research Journal, 1984;21, 435-447.

63. Lepper MR, Henderlong J, Gingras I. 'Understanding the effects of extrinsic rewards on intrinsic motivation - Uses and abuses of meta-analysis: Comment on Deci, Koestner, and Ryan'. Psychological Bulletin, 1999;125, 6, 669-676.

64. Lipsey MW, Wilson DB. 'The Efficacy of Psychological, Educational, and Behavioral Treatment: Confirmation from meta-analysis.' American Psychologist, 1993;48, 12, 1181-1209.

65. Lipsey MW. 'Juvenile delinquency treatment: a meta-analytic inquiry into the variability of effects.' In Cook TD, Cooper H, Cordray DS, Hartmann H, Hedges LV, Light RJ, Louis TA, Mosteller F. (Eds) Meta-analysis for explanation. New York: Russell Sage Foundation, 1992.

66. Maher CG, Sherrington C, Herbert RD, Moseley AM, Elkins M. Reliability of the PEDro scale for rating quality of randomized controlled trials. Physical Therapy, 2003;83(8), 713-721.

67. McGraw KO, Wong SP. 'A Common Language Effect Size Statistic'. Psychological Bulletin, 1992;111, 361-365.

68. McGraw KO. 'Problems with the BESD: a comment on Rosenthal's "How Are We Doing in Soft Psychology". American Psychologist, 1991;46, 1084-6.

69. Methods in Bio-Statistics 6th Edition. 1997: BK Mahajan

70. Miller DC, Salkind NJ. Handbook of research design & social measurement Thousand Oaks, CA: SAGE Publications Ltd. 2002. doi: 10.4135/9781412984386.

71. Mokkink LB, Terwee C, Patrick DL, Alonso J, Stratford PW, Knol DL, et al. The COSMIN checklist for assessing the methodological quality of studies on measurement properties of health status measurement instruments: an international Delphi study. Qual Life Res 2010;19:539e49.

72. Morrison Donald F. Multivariate Statistical Methods, New York: McGraw-Hill, 1967.

73. Mosteller F, Light RJ, Sachs JA. 'Sustained inquiry in education: lessons from skill grouping and class size.' Harvard Educational Review, 1996;66, 797-842.

74. Nassar-McMillan SC, Borders D. Use of Focus Groups in Survey Item Development. The Qualitative Report, 2002;7(1). Retrieved from http://www.nsuworks.nova.edu/tqr/vol7/iss1/3/.

75. Nunnally Jum C. Psychometric Theory, 2nd ed., New York: McGraw-Hill, 1978.

76. Oakes M. Statistical Inference: A Commentary for the Social and Behavioral Sciences. New York: Wiley, 1986.

77. Olejnik S, Algina J. 'Measures of Effect Size for Comparative Studies: Applications, Interpretations and Limitations.' Contemporary Educational Psychology, 2000;25, 241-286.

78. Plano Clark, Vicki L, John W. Creswell. Understanding Research: A Consumer's Guide, Melbourne, Pearson (Merrill), 2009.

79. Portney L, Watkins M, et al. Foundations of clinical research: applications to practice, Prentice Hall Upper Saddle River, NJ, 2000.

80. Rao NSN. Elements of Health Statistics: Tara Publications; 1978.

81. Rosenthal R, Rubin DB. 'A simple, general purpose display of magnitude of experimental effect.' Journal of Educational Psychology, 1982;74, 166-169.

82. Rosenthal R. 'Parametric Measures of Effect Size' in H. Cooper and L.V. Hedges (Eds.). The Handbook of Research Synthesis. New York: Russell Sage Foundation, 1994.

83. Rubin DB. 'Meta-analysis: literature synthesis or effect-size surface estimation.' Journal of Educational Statistics, 1992;17, 4, 363-374.

84. Shymansky JA, Hedges LV, Woodworth G. A reassessment of the effects of inquiry-based science curricula of the 60's on student performance.' Journal of Research in Science Teaching, 1990;27, 127-144.

85. Siegel S. Nonparametric Statistics for the Behavioral Sciences, New York: McGraw-Hill Publishing Co., Inc., 1956.

86. Slavin RE, Madden NA. 'What works for students at risk? A research synthesis.' Educational Leadership, 1989;46(4), 4-13.

87. Smith ML, Glass GV. 'Meta-analysis of research on class size and its relationship to attitudes and instruction.' American Educational Research Journal, 1980;17, 419-433.

88. Snyder P, Lawson S. 'Evaluating Results Using Corrected and Uncorrected Effect Size Estimates.' Journal of Experimental Education, 1993;61, 4, 334-349.

89. Standards of validity and the validity of standards in performance assessment. Messick, Samuel; Educational Measurement: Issues and Practice, Vol 14(4), Win, 1995.

90. Strahan RF. 'Remarks on the Binomial Effect Size Display'. American Psychologist, 1991;46, 1083-4.

91. Tandon BC. Research Methodology in Social Sciences, Allahabad: Chaitanya Publishing House, 1979.

92. Thompson B. 'Common methodology mistakes in educational research, revisited, along with a primer on both effect sizes and the bootstrap.' Invited address presented at the annual meeting of the American Educational Research Association, Montreal, 1999. [Accessed from http://acs.tamu.edu/~bbt6147/aeraad99. htm , January 2000]

93. Tymms P, Merrell C, Henderson B. 'The First Year as School: A Quantitative Investigation of the Attainment and Progress of Pupils'. Educational Research and Evaluation, 1997;3, 2, 101-118.

94. Vincent D, Crumpler M. British Spelling Test Series Manual 3X/Y. Windsor: NFER-Nelson, 1997.

95. Wang MC, Baker ET. 'Mainstreaming programs: Design features and effects. Journal of Special Education, 1986;19, 503-523.

96. Wilcox RR. 'How many discoveries have been lost by ignoring modern statistical methods?'. American Psychologist, 1998;53, 3, 300-314.

97. Wilkinson L. Task Force on Statistical Inference, APA Board of Scientific Affairs. 'Statistical Methods in Psychology Journals: Guidelines and Explanations'. American Psychologist, 1999;54, 8, 594-604.

Index